Every Woman's guide to Cosmetic Surgery

Andrew Skanderowicz FRCS and
Edward Latimer-Sayer FRCS

NEW
HOLLAND

First published in 2007 by New Holland Publishers (UK) Ltd
London • Cape Town • Sydney • Auckland

1 3 5 7 9 10 8 6 4 2

www.newhollandpublishers.com

Garfield House, 86–88 Edgware Road, London W2 2EA, UK
80 McKenzie Street, Cape Town 8001, South Africa
14 Aquatic Drive, Frenchs Forest, NSW 2086, Australia
218 Lake Road, Northcote, Auckland, New Zealand

ISBN: 978 1 84537 702 1

Editorial Director: Jo Hemmings
Editor: Kate Parker
Copy Editor: Naomi Waters
Assistant Editor: Giselle Osborne
Design and cover design: Ian Hughes, Mousemat Design Ltd
Production: Joan Woodroffe

Reproduction by Modern Age Repro House, Hong Kong
Printed and bound by Replika Press PVT Ltd, India

Note: The author and publishers have made every effort to ensure that the
information given in this book is safe and accurate, but they cannot accept
liability for any resulting injury or loss or damage to either property or
person, whether direct or consequential and howsoever arising.

We would like to dedicate this book to our loved ones,

for all the support they have given us in its production.

We would also like to acknowledge the vital role that our

previous patients have had in allowing us to gain the

necessary expertise and experience.

Contents

Foreword

Cosmetic surgery can achieve almost unbelievable results. It has never been so popular and accessible, and celebrity endorsement has made it top of the wish list for not just the rich and famous but for ordinary folk as well.

But whether you are contemplating a simple Botox® treatment to iron out wrinkles, liposuction for troublesome areas of flab, or a more major procedure on your breast or face, it should never be undertaken lightly.

When a patient's expectations are unrealistically high or when inexperienced surgeons, employed by less reputable clinics, are let loose on an unsuspecting public, disappointment or even disaster can ensue.

It is always vital that the right surgery is done for the right reason, on the right patient, by the right surgeon. It is also imperative that sufficient time is devoted to preoperative counselling, so that informed consent can be given and the patient is fully aware of what to expect.

This book, written by two highly respected and professional colleagues of mine, with many years of cosmetic experience behind them, provides a comprehensive overview of everything anyone contemplating cosmetic surgery could ever need to know; not just a basic understanding of the benefits and risks, but a detailed description – in plain English – of the actual procedures themselves.

We live in a world where most media coverage of the subject is either journalistic hype, corporate advertorial or blatant scaremongering. It is difficult to know what to believe.

Every Woman's Guide to Cosmetic Surgery is different. It is the book you certainly can believe and I believe it is an essential read for any woman considering cosmetic surgery.

Dr Hilary Jones

About the Authors

Andrew Skanderowicz FRCS has been practising cosmetic surgery full time since 1982. He has busy practices in London and Dublin and was one of the pioneers of liposuction in the UK, when it was first popularised internationally in the early 1980s. Although Andrew performs all the common cosmetic procedures he has a particular interest in rhinoplasty.

He has held the posts of Academic Secretary and Secretary of the British Association of Cosmetic Surgeons and is currently its President.

Andrew is of the firm opinion that all cosmetic surgery should be entirely controlled by the medical profession without the non-medically qualified counsellors or agents who exploit the speciality and often give it a bad name.

In 1986, Andrew established The Dublin Cosmetic Surgery Centre in Ireland, which was the first of its kind in the country. It was an instant success and today is busier than ever. In 1989, he established The London Cosmetic Surgery Centre, which has recently expanded and moved to bigger premises.

Andrew can be contacted as follows: London: +44 (0)20 7487 5736/ Dublin: +353 (0)1 6611637/www.renewyou.co.uk

Edward Latimer-Sayer FRCS qualified as a medical practitioner in 1971. He left the NHS in 1978 to become a cosmetic surgeon working in full-time private practice. Over the past 28 years, he has personally operated on many thousands of patients. He feels that proper mutual communication between the patient and the surgeon is an essential requirement for successful cosmetic surgery.

He was elected Secretary of the British Association of Cosmetic Surgeons 1993–5 and he is Vice-President of the European Confederation of Aesthetic Surgical Societies. He is frequently consulted by cosmetic-surgery colleagues for advice and information regarding problem patients, and by solicitors to give opinions on the cosmetic surgery performed by other surgeons.

For the past 10 years he has specialised in facelifting, using various techniques, and also secondary (revision) rhinoplasty. He has attended and lectured at many international conferences, and has published articles on various aspects of facelifting. While keeping up-to-date with all the latest developments and techniques, he preserves a healthy sense of scepticism so as to protect his patients from every new gimmick that comes along.

Edward can be contacted via his website: www.latimer-sayer.co.uk, where you can find many 'before and after' photographs of common operations.

Introduction

We have both been in full-time cosmetic-surgery practice for over 25 years. In that time we have performed thousands of procedures. We have always done our utmost to satisfy our patients, and can proudly boast that we have been successful most of the time. However, we would not be telling the truth if we said that absolutely everyone we have ever operated on or treated was completely and utterly satisfied with the results. Any physically invasive procedure on the human body has a risk of complications and unfavourable consequences, even in the best hands. If we were the best surgeons that had ever lived, we would still not satisfy everyone.

Our vast experience has taught us always to be cautious, not to take anything for granted and to be prepared for the unexpected because sooner or later it will happen. Our speciality is never boring, always has something new to teach us and gives us immense job satisfaction.

By pooling our knowledge and experience, we felt it would be of benefit to the general public to write this book – to serve as an authoritative guide to those seriously considering cosmetic surgery, and those who are simply curious about the subject. We have tried to keep it as simple as possible, without the use of incomprehensible medical terminology. At the same time, we have tried to ensure that the reader benefits from all the known facts as well as from our own personal advice and experience.

The number of people undergoing cosmetic surgery has dramatically increased in the last few years. They come from all walks of life and are of all ages. Cosmetic surgery is becoming increasingly socially acceptable, and more and more people are now aware of the benefits. Furthermore, recent advances in the design of implants and surgical and anaesthetic techniques have greatly improved results and shortened the time needed for recovery. Perhaps the most important single reason for the rapid rise in popularity of cosmetic surgery has been the huge media coverage and publicity that this surgical speciality attracts.

With this increase in the popularity of cosmetic surgery it became apparent very quickly that there was a great demand for less invasive treatments for those who were either too apprehensive or squeamish, or those not prepared to undergo the more invasive and extensive procedures. In our opinion some of these less invasive procedures do have benefits. However, many are not as effective or as long lasting as the more traditional and long-established, invasive ones. We have included the more effective ones, which do not necessarily require the skills and expertise of the invasive surgeon.

The aim of cosmetic surgery is to improve a person's external appearance, but it must be stressed that surgery is not an exact science and that the surgeon cannot always precisely deliver what the patient has in mind. It is important to realise at the outset that cosmetic surgery obeys just the same rules as all other branches of surgery. Results cannot therefore be promised or guaranteed, and complications can occasionally occur that are outside the control of the surgeon, no matter how brilliant or experienced he or she is.

The surgical procedures described in this book have been performed successfully thousands of times throughout the world and the vast majority of patients are very happy with the results of their surgery.

Every person is unique. There are many different ways in which a person can be concerned by their appearance and expectations are so individual that this book is not intended to act as a substitute for a consultation with the operating surgeon. There is little doubt that the average person seeking cosmetic surgery today has far higher expectations than before. In order to avoid disappointment, every aspect of a procedure or treatment must be properly explained by the surgeon and thoroughly understood by the patient.

More than in any other field of surgery – because, by definition, cosmetic surgery is rarely a medical necessity – the decision to proceed rests entirely with the client after a detailed discussion with the operating surgeon and a great deal of thought. Every potential patient must be fully aware of the nature of the procedure, the possible or likely result, as well as the potential risks involved.

We encourage potential patients to make a note of any queries which may arise after reading this book and discuss them with their surgeon at a preoperative consultation. Patients cannot always remember everything from that first consultation, so we hope this book can also serve to refresh the patient's mind about what they may have discussed previously with their own surgeon.

Cosmetic surgery is not for everyone. There are many factors that may render a person unsuitable. We hope that after reading this book, the unsuitable candidate will desist from seeking cosmetic surgery and will not begin the process that will lead to getting on to an operating table. Not only will this save a lot of money, but it will also prevent certain disappointment, for the surgeon as well as them.

PART ONE
ABOUT COSMETIC SURGERY

A surgical operation is a controlled injury and the body reacts to it like it does to any injury. Cosmetic surgery is not just about undergoing a surgical procedure, however. Before any patient is subjected to the physical injury of an operation, many other factors have to be considered. Indeed, we are firmly of the opinion that the preoperative considerations and preparatory events leading up to the big day when the surgeon makes the first incision, are equally if not *more* important, than the actual operative procedure.

Many people who undergo cosmetic surgery have never been in hospital before and are understandably frightened by the prospect. Some are more afraid of having a general anaesthetic than undergoing the operation itself. Fear of the unknown is natural and forever present in the field of surgery.

It is hoped that this part of the book will alleviate any worries and fears that an apprehensive patient may have. This part deals with the basic essentials necessary to comprehend and appreciate, in a realistic and balanced manner, all the factors which lead up to an elective cosmetic operation. It encompasses such topics as suitability for surgery, choosing a surgeon, preoperative considerations, admission to a clinic or hospital, the anaesthetic, possible postoperative complications and expectations.

A fully informed patient is far more likely to be less apprehensive about undergoing surgery, be less nervous on the day of surgery and more likely to accept and come to terms with the possible, common postoperative events that are likely to be encountered. A fully informed patient is forewarned and therefore forearmed to face any possible eventuality. This can only be of benefit to the patient (as well as the surgeon and his staff).

The Concept of Beauty

Since the dawn of history men and women have attempted to modify their appearance to comply with the cultural standards of the era. There are many philosophical theories to explain this concept but it doesn't take a genius to work out that a physically attractive man and woman are more likely to get married or find a partner (as they are more sought after by the opposite sex), get better jobs and generally be more confident and successful.

Although it is not possible to define beauty easily – it varies with different cultures and is dependent on the eye of the beholder – there are certain physical characteristics that are significant for the overall ideal concept of beauty.

It is commonly said that the 'ideal woman' has a small chin, delicate jaw, large lips, small nose, prominent cheekbones, large and widely spaced eyes and a waist-to-hip ratio of 0.7. The 'ideal man' is tall, has rugged macho features – rectangular face and chin, deep-set eyes, heavy brow, large straight nose in proportion to the size of the face – and a waist-to-hip ratio of 0.9.

It is common for men and women to try to accentuate the differences between them. For instance, women are generally less hairy than men, so go to a lot of trouble to make sure that they are even less so. They also have softer skin than men and there is a huge industry devoted to selling women products that will soften the skin and protect it from becoming weather beaten and therefore more 'masculine'.

Interestingly, sexual attractiveness and the concept of beauty are not necessarily the same thing. Attractiveness for a woman usually means that she looks healthy and is of a fertile age. When a man says a woman is attractive and 'sexy' he is observing the signs of possible fertility. Every 'Miss World' who has ever won the contest has had the waist-to-hip ratio of 0.7. Research has shown that women who have this ratio are more fertile than those that don't.

When a woman finds a young man attractive she is often seeing the signs caused by testosterone, the hormone that makes a man masculine (and more fertile). If she finds an older man attractive, she is (possibly subconsciously) seeing a man who may be able to provide for her and any children she might have.

Detailed and accurate measurements of facial features and angles have tried to add a more scientific element to the concept of beauty. When these measurements are analysed and applied to different ethnic groups, those considered to be good looking or beautiful comply with universal scientific concepts of beauty. Thus, in the main, a particular ethnic beauty will still be considered attractive by the majority of any other ethnic group.

Many studies have stressed the importance of facial symmetry. No human face is exactly symmetrical, but marked asymmetry – beyond what is considered normal – is not usually considered to be beautiful. This is probably because of the association of good symmetry with good health.

Asymmetry is sometimes caused by sleeping on one side more than the other. Most people prefer to sleep on one particular side, a pattern that is established early in life. Babies tend to sleep a lot and grow while they are asleep; the side that is on the pillow doesn't grow as much as the uppermost side. This means that, when an adult has one side of their face that is smaller than the other, it is possible to guess on which side they prefer to sleep.

At the same time it must be stressed that although facial appearance is a very important parameter when considering the concept of beauty, other bodily features are also important. These will include height, shape, amount of fat distribution on the body, breast size and shape, skin quality and so forth. A man or woman may not be particularly facially attractive but have a near perfect figure, and vice versa.

Of course, you have to add a person's personality, or 'inner beauty' into the equation. Plenty of beautiful people get married, only to separate soon after. Physical attractiveness does not necessarily guarantee a long-term relationship, and in some ways can even detract from it.

Whatever may be analysed by philosophers and experts regarding the concept of beauty – and much has been said and written on the subject – the truth remains that many people are never satisfied with what Nature gave them in terms of their physical appearance.

We have learned from experience that even stunningly attractive people find fault in their appearance, often exaggerating their problem when it may seem negligible to the average onlooker. It is difficult to explain the reasons for this, but it is possible that this particular group of people set themselves very high standards from an early age and are so preoccupied with their appearance that, the moment they perceive a deterioration, they immediately seek help.

Learned psychologists will attempt to explain this phenomenon as a personality flaw. Many psychologists still denigrate cosmetic surgery as unnecessary and attempt to explain any strong reaction to a blemish as a deep-rooted mental aberration. But, despite all the complex jargon and scientific research conducted in an attempt to explain it, they are unable to offer a simple treatment or cure that will satisfy those afflicted with an abnormal obsessional disorder pertaining to their physical appearance. In our experience, attempting to convince a patient that her nose is pretty when she is convinced it is not, simply does not work.

Most people we meet in our practice every day are perfectly normal individuals who simply dislike a particular part of their anatomy, and would like it improved. In the vast majority of cases, the results of surgery are very successful and the patient resumes a normal lifestyle with renewed confidence.

There is no doubt that there are those who will never be happy with their appearance no matter what. These people can usually, but not always, be spotted by the experienced surgeon, and the only ethical response is to refuse them treatment (see 'Is Cosmetic Surgery *Really* For You?', pages 68–71). The surgeon may then refer the patient for counselling, really the only alternative when surgery will undoubtedly prove unsatisfactory.

How successful counselling may eventually prove will depend on the expertise of the counsellor and the seriousness of the person's condition. One thing is certain – no amount of counselling can remove a physical blemish! As to whether someone can be persuaded that they do not really have a problem, when for years they have despaired of their particular blemish, is a matter for debate. We have certainly not encountered a case where this has happened. Conversely, however, we have both seen patients who have been cured of psychiatric problems by having successful cosmetic surgery.

It is hard not to feel pressure to look one's best. Media coverage constantly exposes women to pictures of beautiful women, and advertising for beauty-enhancement products. Add to this any active criticism of a blemish an individual may have received from those around them, and a person can feel surrounded by reminders of their physical imperfections. Realistically, adults are no different from children in this respect. We have even encountered patients who were not ridiculed as children, but only when they became adults. All this leads to an ever-increasing sense of self-deprecation.

Early Childhood

Problems can start early in life if classroom bullying and teasing is rife. A common example is the child with protruding ears. Such teasing can lead to serious consequences for both child and parents. The child will detest going to school, become withdrawn, unhappy and depressed. His or her early developmental progress at school may be seriously compromised. The parents will suffer likewise, very often at a loss as to how to solve the problem.

Ears are fully developed by the age of five and a simple operation (see 'Correction of Protruding Ears', pages 126–129) at that stage can alleviate a lot of potential psychological damage in the future.

Adolescence

The next stage is the adolescent going through puberty. This is the time when many teenagers experience the onset of acne, which may be quite disfiguring. Other problems that occur at this time include problems with the development of secondary sexual characteristics e.g. breast-development in girls. This is often a time of turmoil for many teenagers who constantly strive to look their best and comply with the latest fashion trends in order not to be the odd one out.

We are now operating on more younger people than before. Schoolgirls will seek breast enlargement to avoid ridicule by their peers. Some will refuse to attend sports activities because it means undressing in front of classmates and changing into sports kit. Nose reshaping is also becoming more frequent in teenagers, as is liposuction. However, we do not feel that cosmetic surgery should generally be offered to teenagers unless the problem is particularly severe.

Early Adulthood

At the age of 18, most females have reached full physical maturity. They stop growing and have fully developed sexual characteristics, facial features and body shape. This is the time when a general overhaul of aesthetic appearance takes serious priority.

In the majority, if adolescence precluded seeking or establishing a relationship with the opposite sex because of the usual restrictions, early adulthood, with its new freedoms, can make up for the shortfall. At this time most will be seeking to look their best in order to attract a partner.

Cosmetic surgeons will see patients in their young adulthood who will request nearly all the commonly available procedures, apart from those specific to reversing the aging process.

Middle Age

This is the next category of self-referral for cosmetic surgery. By this time most women will have had children. The early signs of facial aging will also be taking their toll.

A woman might complain of smaller, drooping breasts; a loose, flabby abdomen, and varicose or thread veins as a result of childbearing. The more children she has had, the more pronounced the problem. In addition she will probably have put on weight and be concerned about her facial appearance, particularly if she has been a heavy smoker for many years. She may therefore be seeking facial fillers and Botox®, as well as surgery.

Over the years, we have observed that many women request a facelift at the age of 50 and satisfy themselves that by doing this at that age it will last them until old age when they will not be concerned about their appearance. Many do not realise that they will still strive to look their best even at 70 because mentally they will probably feel the same as they did at 50. We often see women coming back ten years later for a repeat procedure.

Old Age

The majority of patients at this age are women who are mostly concerned with facial and eyelid aging. In addition many will request facial fillers and Botox® even though at that age fillers and Botox® will have very limited beneficial effect. By this stage many will not be physically fit for surgery or not even be particularly concerned about their appearance, electing instead to grow old gracefully. Only those who are in good health will be operated on.

Conclusion

Although the concept of beauty is difficult to define precisely, one thing is for certain: with ever-improving and developing technologies, most women can rest assured that a great deal can be achieved to enhance their aesthetic appearance and thereby bring increased self satisfaction and self confidence.

The perception of beauty is ultimately a matter of personal taste and opinion. One thing is for certain – if we all had the identical concept of beauty all men would be attracted to the same women and vice versa, leaving many disappointed individuals overlooked. It is patently obvious that we have been designed to hold diverse views and opinions on what we find beautiful so that the human race can continue to procreate and survive.

The History of Cosmetic Surgery in the UK

If we define cosmetic surgery as surgery that alters physical appearance, then nearly all human cultures from the Stone Age onwards seem to have adopted practices that altered the appearance of members of the tribe. In Kenya, marks on the face were made by cutting the skin and then rubbing in earth so that the resulting scar was wide and visible. The idea was that a member of any particular tribe was instantly recognisable. Many tribesmen and women had bones or other objects forced through noses and earlobes. They did this, or had this done to them, for the age-old reason that they wanted to fit in and look like other members of their society. This is pretty much the same reason why the majority of cosmetic-surgery patients today seek surgery.

Although it is true to say that cosmetic surgery is still a relatively new speciality in the UK, it dates back for centuries. The beginnings of eyelid surgery can be traced back to the 10th century in Arabia. The first record of a facelift was in the early 1900s, although it is not known who attempted the very first one.

As early as 600 BC, the first evidence of nose reconstruction (rhinoplasty) was recorded. By the end of the 1st century, rhinoplasty was common as a result of the uncivilised practice of cutting off the noses and lips of one's enemies. By the 16th century, noses were reconstructed after being severed in duels by using flaps of upper arm skin: necessity was the mother of invention!

Otoplasty (correction of protruding ears) was described in the 1850s, although there is some evidence to show that it was performed much earlier. The first breast reduction can be traced back to the 15th century, while the first silicone implant for breast augmentation was performed in

1963. Prior to that, breasts were enlarged using dermal (deep layer of skin) grafts and even injecting liquid silicone, a practice that was short lived because of the disastrous consequences. The injection of liquid paraffin was also tried at various times since 1889, but the results were poor and the complications horrendous.

The most modern revolutionary cosmetic surgical procedure dates back to the early 1970s when surgeons in Switzerland described for the first time a technique for sucking out fat. The initial trials were not a total success because of the frequency of postoperative complications, notably seromas (large accumulations of fluid under the skin), which took a long time to absorb, and skin depressions. In 1977, a French surgeon, Gerard Illouz, perfected the technique by using a blunt cannula (surgical tube) connected to a high negative pressure vacuum pump.

In most countries of the world, when a doctor qualifies as a specialist he sets about establishing a practice. There are various professional ways to do this. The usual way is to inform all of his colleagues that he is available to receive referrals relevant to his speciality, and he also sets about telling as many people as possible what he does and how to find him. Hopefully, sooner or later his reputation grows and his practice increases. Some specialists buy into already established practices as a junior partner and in many countries it is possible to buy a practice from someone who is retiring.

After the inception of the NHS in Great Britain in 1948, the system became quite different. It was only possible to set up as a specialist once one had been appointed a consultant. The supply of consultant posts was very restricted, so a doctor only became a consultant when a post became vacant. There were always very many more trained doctors than there were posts available.

Doctors who became consultants under this system claim that only the best were chosen, but this was not always the case, as many doctors became disillusioned and either gave up hospital medicine or emigrated. It also meant that, in Britain, many fully trained doctors could not get consultant posts and remained so-called junior doctors well into their 40s. This led to the concept that doctors who trained in the NHS needed 14 years or so after qualification to become adept in their speciality. The rest of the world did not believe this and overseas specialists became fully qualified at a much younger age.

The reason for the late appointment of consultants in the NHS was the bottleneck created by the lack of posts available. The training of junior doctors was generally on-the-job training, in an ad hoc fashion, more li an apprenticeship. Often there was no formal training; a junior doctor had to serve his time and hope that a consultant post became available when he was sufficiently senior.

When the authors of this book were junior doctors in the NHS in the 1970s there was no formal training in cosmetic surgery. There still isn't really, because very few purely cosmetic operations are performed in NHS hospitals. Nearly all cosmetic surgery is done in the private sector. Both the authors left the NHS and gained their training by following senior surgeons who had busy private practices.

Plastic surgery was established as a speciality only relatively recently, after the Second World War. Plastic surgeons claimed cosmetic surgery as part of their speciality, but in reality many different types of surgeon have been performing cosmetic surgery for over 150 years. It is not true that plastic surgeons are the only ones who are fully qualified, as they claim, to carry it out. Their own training programme has only recently embraced cosmetic procedures. They spend most of their time carrying out operations on burns, malformations and injuries and their training reflects this. It is quite common even today for a plastic surgeon to become a fully qualified specialist with virtually no experience in cosmetic surgery.

There is little common ground between the usual NHS plastic-surgery patient and those seeking a cosmetic operation. Cosmetic patients are generally much more exacting in their expectations than those who need cancer surgery or skin grafting for burns.

There used to be a total prohibition on any form of advertising by doctors. This was designed to protect vulnerable patients from blandishments from unscrupulous doctors. In reality, it protected and controlled the referral system of private patients by GPs to hospital consultants. Up until the 1970s it was never imagined that this 'in-house' system could or would be challenged by anyone. But challenged it was, by a group of entrepreneurs who took advantage of a legal loophole that allowed non-medical people to set up independent private medical services, which then employed surgeons and anaesthetists.

These entrepreneurs had only one thought in mind; medical ethics were certainly not high on the agenda. They were not regulated by any ethical body, and were therefore allowed to publicly promote and advertise medical services in the media. As a result private medical services began to be established offering abortions, medical screening and cosmetic surgery.

Some unscrupulous individuals saw this as a passport to making easy money and established some of the first cosmetic surgery clinics in the 1970s. Many employed hard-sell tactics and adopted the attitude that they were beyond reproach as any mishap could easily be blamed on the doctor. Therefore, they would refuse to take any responsibility in the event of a problem. These individuals quickly gained control of the cosmetic-surgery industry.

Unfortunately, many doctors did not approve of cosmetic surgery in any form and refused to refer their patients. This meant that many patients had no way of finding a surgeon who performed cosmetic surgery unless they contacted one of these clinics. Since that time the number of these clinics and establishments in the UK has grown enormously, particularly since 2001. Every major town and city has several different providers in competition with one another.

As a result of the activities of commercial clinics, the rules on medical advertising have now been very considerably relaxed and numbers of doctors appear in the media hawking their skills. Often they are the same doctors who only a few years ago accused surgeons who worked for commercial clinics of being unethical.

Advertising is still generally disapproved of by most of the profession. However, in Britain today, the majority of cosmetic operations are performed by doctors working for commercial clinics. These clinics have a financial imperative to carry out as many operations as possible and, certainly in the past, dubious methods were used to get patients to sign up. It is however commercial suicide to run an unethical clinic and most, but by no means all, clinics these days treat their patients with consideration and skill. There is still a risk, however, that a vulnerable patient may meet a salesman or woman paid on commission who will say virtually anything in order to get them to undergo treatment.

Whatever the criticism of cosmetic surgery in the past, one thing is patently obvious: in expert hands it is extremely successful and has transformed the lives of many people for the better. It is here to stay and is growing very quickly.

We hope that the information in this book will give patients the knowledge to make good judgements about whether to have surgery or not and protect them from the more unethical fringes of the cosmetic-surgery industry.

The British Association of Cosmetic Surgeons (BACS)

Cosmetic surgery is a relatively new surgical speciality in the UK and is not readily available in the National Health Service (NHS). Up until quite recently there was relatively little interest in this speciality. It was even frowned upon by many medical practitioners who regarded cosmetic surgery as unnecessary and frivolous.

Because there was little to offer in the way of surgical expertise in cosmetic surgery in the late 1970s and early 1980s in the UK, a group of surgeons, from various surgical specialties, inaugurated the British Association of Cosmetic Surgeons (BACS) in 1980. What united them was their interest in cosmetic surgery as a speciality in its own right.

The British Association of Cosmetic Surgeons was established to promote the study and practice of cosmetic surgery, to act as a forum for the exchange of information and ideas among its members and to promote and maintain the highest standards in this speciality. The Association has a defined Constitution as well as a strict Code of Practice, which all members must abide by at all times.

The Association has grown over the years but has never lost sight of its initial aims. The entry criteria, which have to be satisfied by all new members, are strict, and membership is an honour. Full membership is only granted to those who are Fellows of one of the Royal Colleges of Surgeons (FRCS), or hold the equivalent European qualification and have proven competence in cosmetic surgery. Competence is assessed by already established members of the Association who report their findings and opinions to the membership for final approval before admission to the Association.

In recent years the Association has opened its membership to include Associate Members. Associate Members are qualified medical practitioners but do not necessarily hold the same qualifications as Full Members. These practitioners engage in the regular practice of cosmetic procedures, but often those less complex than those performed by full members e.g. Hair Transplantation, Laser Skin Surgery or Thread Vein Treatment.

The Association holds regular clinical meetings and encourages members to travel widely to attend seminars and conferences to keep up to date with progress in this speciality. All surgeons have to audit their work and undergo regular revalidation under the auspices of the General Medical Council and Royal Colleges.

We would stress that the British Association of Cosmetic Surgeons is not the only association or group of medical practitioners that practice cosmetic surgery in the UK. The British Association of Cosmetic Surgeons was however the first group of surgeons to be established in the UK, whose main dedication was to enhance the practice of cosmetic surgery and whose members performed cosmetic surgery full-time. There are other groups of surgeons and doctors, generally drawn from narrow fields, such as Ear, Nose and Throat (ENT), Maxillofacial and Plastic Surgery.

The BACS Code of Practice

Before admission to the Association each member must agree to abide by the Association's Code of Practice at all times. The Code does not purport to be a complete Code of Ethics of conduct and the Council of the Association specifically reserves the right to amend the code as and when it deems appropriate.

1. All patients seeking cosmetic surgery will receive thorough and meticulous preoperative counselling with full information both verbal and written as is necessary for a full understanding of the procedure and its complications. In addition, patients will be asked to confirm in writing that they have received and understood such information.

2. The surgeons must use their best endeavours to make sure that if non-medically trained counsellors (or any other counsellors who are not members of the medical profession) are imparting advice to patients, then that advice must not interfere/conflict with the advice that has or may be imparted to the patient by the surgeon. The

regulation applies to all preoperative advice, postoperative advice and treatment. Where the surgeon becomes aware that there has been any interference/conflicting advice, then he/she must take immediate steps to re-affirm his/her advice to the patient.

3. Adequate time should be allowed between preoperative consultation and the operation in order to give the patient every opportunity to consider carefully all the facts pertaining to treatment.

4. The Association recognises that adequate time may vary depending upon the type of surgery requested. The Association recognises that some patients may wish to have the operation on the same day as the consultation and, if this is the case, then the patient shall be asked to sign a form stating that the Surgeon has recommended that there should be an adequate lapse of time between the consultation and the operation, that the patient has understood the advice and has instructed the Surgeon to proceed on the same day as the consultation.

5. In circumstances whereby the Surgeon becomes aware that a patient may require an operation on the same day as the consultation then he/she must use his/her best endeavours to send to the patient all relevant information and literature pertaining to his/her operation/ treatment, some time before the consultation.

6. Surgery must only be performed in places that are properly equipped and staffed for such surgery. There are some clinics and organisations recommended by BACS, and Members must not carry out cosmetic surgery in clinics or organisations that are not on the recommended list. The list is constantly reviewed and updated and a Member may approach the Council at any stage and ask for a particular organisation/clinic to be placed on the recommended list. Provided three Members of the Council approve then that organisation/clinic will be added to the recommended list.

7. All members must ensure that any literature/documentation that he/she would normally impart to his/her patients relating to the Surgeon's speciality is constantly reviewed and, where appropriate, updated. All members will, pursuant to a written request from the Council, produce copies of the aforementioned literature/documentation for inspection by the Council within 14 days of a written request.

8. All members must only perform cosmetic surgery in the approved module(s) for which they have been admitted as Members of the Association. If a member wishes to extend his Membership to cover any other approved cosmetic surgery module in respect of which he/she has not been admitted as a Member then he/she must make the appropriate application to the Membership Committee to extend his/her category of Membership.

Cosmetic Surgery and the Media

When cosmetic surgery first started to become popular in the UK in the early 1980s it attracted very limited media coverage. Articles in magazines and newspapers were based on information from the USA and would only appear every few months. In total contrast, in the last few years a day doesn't go by without some mention of cosmetic surgery in the media. Without doubt this surgical speciality attracts more media coverage than any other type of surgery.

Significant amounts of cosmetic surgery were done in the past, but patients tended to be quite secretive about having had it done and tried to avoid publicity. Also, there were very severe restrictions placed on doctors regarding advertising. If any doctor allowed his name to appear in print he risked being struck off and losing his livelihood. This has all changed now. Many doctors advertise openly, and some blatantly seek any publicity in order to increase their practices.

A word must also be said about the volume of advertising and advertorials in the media concerning clinics. Many clinics spend a lot of money with public relations (PR) companies to promote their services in the media. The more successful PR companies have a direct working relationship with editors of popular magazines and newspapers and can arrange for favourable articles to be published about their particular establishment. Quite often, media articles featuring wildly ecstatic patients are simply advertisements for the clinics concerned. We urge caution in believing everything you read, as there are some establishments that are extremely ruthless in the way they conduct themselves, and in our opinion they give cosmetic surgery a bad name.

It is easy to understand why the media publishes so many articles on the subject. The idea of anyone subjecting their body to physical assault in pursuit of enhancing their appearance attracts much criticism and controversy but, above all, the huge curiosity of the general public.

Nowadays, the back pages of both women's and men's magazines are full of advertisements for cosmetic surgery. In addition, television programmes on enhancing appearance by cosmetic surgery regularly appear on our screens.

From the point of view of the cosmetic surgeon, this media coverage is a double-edged sword. On the one hand, it increases the number of people seeking surgery, but on the other, the editorialising of many of these programmes can often lead to false hopes and ideas, making this a potential banana-skin situation for the surgeon. For this reason, most cosmetic surgeons who have been practising this speciality for many years will agree that patient expectations today are far higher than ever before.

Not all media reports about cosmetic surgery are favourable. Very often stories are incorrectly reported or overly dramatised to make them appear more unfavourable than they really are. The reason is simple. The more dramatic, controversial and unfavourable the report is, the more attention it will attract. Serious adverse incidents are, actually, very rare.

Government guidelines are now in place with respect to all medical specialities in an attempt to keep adverse incidents to a minimum. In addition, more stringent controls are being exercised regarding the suitability and qualifications of practitioners who perform these procedures. It is undoubtedly true to say that the vast majority of cosmetic operations and procedures are very successful and prospective patients should not be unduly apprehensive.

General
Considerations

Cosmetic surgery can be defined as 'that branch of surgery whose primary aim is the enhancement of the non-pathological external appearance of a patient'.

In cosmetic surgery perfection is the aim, rarely the achievement. What may be deemed an acceptable result by one patient may be totally unacceptable to another. The realistic aim of cosmetic surgery therefore is to improve the appearance of a particular feature or deformity with the intention of achieving increased self-satisfaction and self-confidence.

Those expecting a miracle or a result that is outside the realms of surgical possibility will doubtless be disappointed. A particular surgeon may be unable to match what a patient has in mind regarding the final appearance. On occasions it may transpire that the goal of the patient would not actually suit him or her, or prove to be disappointing, even if attained.

The successful result of any cosmetic surgical procedure thus depends not only on the skill and experience of the surgeon, but also on a number of factors outside the surgeon's direct control. These factors include the patient's general health, age, skin texture, bone structure, healing properties, and the expectations of the patient. These can all influence the final result.

It is possible for complications to occur that in the short term can spoil a result. Complications occur in all branches of medicine and surgery, and are often outside the control of the medical practitioner. Occasionally, a patient may be directly responsible for causing a complication either through carelessness or not following postoperative instructions.

The success or failure of any cosmetic surgical procedure therefore is measured by one factor and one factor only, namely: 'Is the patient happy with the result?' Independent opinions count for nothing if the patient is dissatisfied.

Although a trained and experienced cosmetic surgeon is a highly qualified medical practitioner, he is not a magician, and is limited by the materials at his disposal. A person who is of moderate attractiveness cannot be turned into a ravishing supermodel by a nose-reshape operation, for example!

Not every prospective patient will be accepted for surgery. Sometimes it is in the patient's best interests to be refused surgery, especially if the result could turn out to be less than satisfactory or, worse still, turn out to be worse than the previous situation. This can occasionally occur.

At the consultation a good surgeon will attempt to assess the patient psychologically as well as physically. This is to help him or her decide if the expected or usual result of the procedure is likely to please the patient. On rare occasions a cosmetic surgeon may refer a patient for a psychiatric opinion before deciding whether to operate. Cosmetic surgery is not a panacea or cure-all for all of life's problems.

The ideal patient must be sufficiently self-motivated to undergo cosmetic surgery. If the desire for cosmetic surgery has been initiated by the 'encouragement' or persistence of a friend, relative or spouse, the end result is more likely to be a disappointment for patient and surgeon alike. It is difficult enough to satisfy and please one patient, let alone their partner and friends as well.

It is extremely unusual to encounter a patient who is not nervous or apprehensive about undergoing cosmetic surgery. This is only natural. Every surgical procedure, even a simple one such as a tooth extraction, entails some degree of risk. There may be complications, and the results may not match expectations.

Seeking Advice – Finding a Surgeon

The British Association of Cosmetic Surgeons (BACS) suggests that patients can find a surgeon by:

1. Contacting the British Association of Cosmetic Surgeons directly.
2. Seeking a referral from their General Practitioner.
3. Getting a recommendation from another patient.
4. Contacting a clinic that advertises to the public.

Contacting the British Association of Cosmetic Surgeons

A list of recommended cosmetic surgeons can be found on the BACS website: www.b-a-c-s.co.uk. These surgeons will all be members or associate members of the BACS (see pages 24–27).

Most surgeons also have their own websites, which can be accessed from the Association's website. Prospective patients are thus able to find out more about a particular surgeon and/or procedure before making contact.

The General Practitioner

This is the system of referral advocated by the General Medical Council (GMC). It dates back from well before the inception of the NHS, when it was considered unethical for a consultant to accept private patients unless they were directly referred by their GP. This was designed to stop unscrupulous consultants touting for patients and treating them inappropriately. However, many patients wishing to undergo cosmetic surgery prefer that their GP is not informed or aware of their intentions. There are many reasons for this.

Many patients are simply too shy or embarrassed to approach their GP for fear of being ridiculed or discouraged from treatment. Some do not wish to burden their overworked GP with a problem involving an element of vanity when he is already so busy with more essential medical problems. Some patients may have already seen their GP, who told them not to have any treatment, and so they would like a second opinion. Others may have been referred by their GP to a surgeon with whom they did not have a rapport and they would like to see someone else.

Many fear that their intentions will be made public because of the nature of the referral system. This necessarily involves the GP's staff who they fear may divulge their secret to others in their community.

Some patients admit to not knowing their GP and would prefer to bypass him altogether. Others are not registered with a GP. Some have openly admitted that they have little trust or faith in their GP and would not contemplate approaching him with such a delicate, personal and private problem.

Although more and more GPs are aware of the benefits that cosmetic surgery can offer and are entirely sympathetic and helpful, there are still a number who are less enthusiastic and who strongly try to dissuade any prospective patients.

Most cosmetic surgeons get very few referrals from GPs.

Recommendation from Another Patient

This is arguably the best and surest way of being referred to a surgeon who has at least proved that he/she is competent at performing the procedure. Most surgeons who do not advertise get the majority of their new patients by referrals from their old patients.

The drawback here is that most patients will not openly or freely admit to undergoing cosmetic surgery, so a prospective patient may not know whether any of their friends and acquaintances has had any surgery.

Clinics that Advertise to the Public

In recent years there has been a huge increase in the number of clinics, establishments and so-called advisory centres offering cosmetic surgery to the public. Many such places are run by non-medically qualified persons who regard it as a quick way of making easy money.

The reason why these establishments have increased in number over the years is that, until quite recently, it was an offence for medical practitioners to advertise their services and expertise to the general public. This could result in the practitioner being struck off the medical register.

It was, however, perfectly legal for a non-medically qualified person to set up a limited company offering cosmetic-surgery services. This company could employ the services of a surgeon and anaesthetist as long as their names were not made public.

Thankfully, with the changes in GMC guidelines, the public is now able to get direct access to the surgeons, and therefore have a greater choice in selecting the one they wish to perform their surgery or treatment.

The BACS advises anyone approaching a clinic that advertises to the public to make sure they see the operating surgeon at a preoperative consultation well in advance of the day of surgery. If the surgeon is not a BACS member, they should make sure they are treated according to, or along similar lines to, the BACS Code of Practice (see pages 25–27). In addition, it is important to find out about the surgeon's experience, qualifications, and proof of previous procedures performed (e.g. pre- and post-operative photographs of the surgeon's work, although it would be extremely difficult to prove beyond doubt that these were in fact photographs of his/her work), and to see as many testimonials from previous patients as possible. (See 'The Preoperative Consultation', pages 42–45.)

We also recommend that patients only be seen by the operating surgeon and not by any other party. Many clinics employ so-called 'counsellors' – often non-medically qualified sales people – to entice people into undergoing surgery. We strongly feel that such a practice is dangerous and can easily lead to patients being given misleading information, which can cause problems later on. Cosmetic surgery is a very personal and private undertaking and depends on a good patient-doctor relationship, without the involvement of any other party. Some commercial clinics are indeed well run and employ competent surgeons who successfully carry out a large number of cosmetic operations.

Cosmetic Surgery Abroad

There are an increasing number of adverts promoting cosmetic surgery abroad, from Eastern Europe to as far away as South Africa and the USA. Some adverts tempt prospective patients by suggesting they combine their surgery with a holiday. The key to persuading patients is the lower cost.

In many countries the cost of living is far lower than in the UK. Hospital and doctors fees are much lower as is the cost of insurance. These factors combine to offer a prospective patient a 'better financial deal'.

It would be professionally unethical for us to criticise or denigrate in any way the practice of cosmetic surgery outside the UK. Indeed, there is no doubt that some establishments abroad offer excellent facilities and the services of perfectly competent surgeons. However, many simply do not. Moreover, as described below, going for surgery abroad can expose you to further risks that you would not encounter if you stayed in the UK.

We have both seen victims of poor and incompetent surgery performed outside the UK. Invariably the unfortunate victim has little, if any, course for redress. Whereas the average cosmetic procedure will cost more in the UK than in many places abroad, one reassuring factor is that in the event of a problem or complication the patient is within easy reach of the hospital and the surgeon who can deal with it promptly and efficiently.

Agents who organise these trips abroad will try to persuade you that any complication will be dealt with. But complications and problems can occur long after you have returned home. What then? Do you then return overseas, or do you try and find a surgeon in the UK willing to take on some other surgeon's problems?

Any competent surgeon, including those practising abroad, will realise that if a patient has travelled a long way to come and see them it is necessary to keep complications down to a minimum. In order to do this, the surgery offered will tend to be more conservative. This could mean that you will achieve less from the operation than if you had seen a more local surgeon.

We stress throughout this book that the initial consultation is the most important part of the treatment process. If you have travelled thousands of miles and more or less booked the operation before even meeting your surgeon, then you are committed, even if only psychologically, to having an operation before all the pros and cons have been explained to you. We feel this is extremely unsafe, and in some cases could lead to having inappropriate surgery. This would be true even for ethical, well-run establishments. In addition to this there are those establishments who will put significant pressure on patients to go ahead against their misgivings once they are caught up in the process and a long way from family and friends who might advise them differently.

The average cost of any cosmetic surgical procedure in the UK is less than the cost of running a motorcar for a year. If you do your homework properly you should manage to find a competent surgeon in your locality and be assured of a good service, without having to pay over the odds.

In summary therefore we do not recommend that you go abroad for your surgery. Do so at your own risk.

Risk Factors Common to All Operations

This chapter deals with those postoperative complications that can occasionally occur with *any* surgical procedure. Complications, which are peculiar, specific or unique to a particular procedure, are discussed in more detail in the appropriate chapter.

The human body is a very complex entity. Despite our current knowledge, we are still only scratching the surface with our understanding of the many intricate mechanisms of its functions and behaviour. We have limited understanding and therefore limited control over the complicated healing process that starts once we down tools.

We rely on the intricate biological, physiological and immunological systems to interact in a controlled and synchronised manner to heal the tissues and give a pleasing cosmetic result with the minimum of scarring or tell-tale signs of surgery. We expect our bodies to do all this despite the magnitude of the physical assault inflicted by the surgery.

The complex mechanism of the healing process is usually the patient's best friend. If all goes according to plan, an area that has been operated on will heal quickly with the minimum of bruising and swelling, leaving a thin scar, barely visible to the naked eye.

On the other hand, the opposite can occur, through no fault of the surgeon, and the operated area may become excessively bruised with permanent pigmentation, persistent swelling or thickening of tissues and a very visible disfiguring scar. At worst, the postoperative appearance may be more disliked by the patient than the preoperative. Revision surgery may be required in an attempt to improve the final result. Thankfully this doesn't happen very often in experienced hands but, when it does, it understandably causes the patient and surgeon concern.

As mentioned previously, every surgical procedure carries a risk, even if performed by the world's best surgeon. It is therefore important for everyone who is contemplating cosmetic surgery to be fully aware of the possible complications that may occasionally occur. This will lessen the psychological trauma and disappointment should anything go wrong.

Nervous patients may be unhappy to take the risk of surgery once they have been informed of all the possible consequences. Bolder ones may be perfectly happy to proceed. In either case, it is the patient's decision, and an ethical surgeon has a duty to give a balanced account of all the risks. In conventional surgery, a surgeon may well try to persuade a patient to have an operation because he believes it is in their medical interests to go ahead. The benefits to their physical health may well outweigh any risks. This is never the case in cosmetic surgery. By definition, it is not medically essential. Thus the patient alone must choose whether they wish to expose themselves to the risks of their procedure. Some patients find it difficult to translate numerical probabilities into factors that affect their decisions on a daily basis. For example, people who truly appreciate the chances of winning the lottery don't waste their money on a ticket!

Most of the complications that are described in this book only happen to a very few, unlucky patients. Indeed, cosmetic surgery is safer and more predictable than conventional surgery, mainly because the patients are healthy – or should be – before the operation. Serious postoperative complications are rare and, if they do occur, further surgery will often rectify or improve the result.

In order to appreciate why complications are unpredictable or indeed occur at all, we must appreciate that every human being has a unique genetic profile. Our genetic profile ultimately controls our health and the way we react to a given set of outside influences or stimuli. It also controls the way our healing process reacts and behaves. Flaws can sometimes occur in the healing process and can predispose to a poor result.

Scars

All surgical incisions heal by producing a scar. To make scars less obvious the surgeon tries to make any necessary incisions where they will not easily be seen, such as in natural skin folds or inside the hairline. It is wrong to think that scars will be invisible or that they will completely fade to nothing in time. The term 'invisible scar' should never be used. Wound healing is an extremely complex, biochemical process involving many variables. For this reason the final results of healing cannot be accurately predicted.

Once an incision is made and sutured (stitched) the surgeon has little control over the healing process.

Most scars will look worse (red and raised) for some time after the operation before they mature and become pale and level with the surrounding skin. In general, scars take six to 18 months to mature (in some cases, they can take longer). There will always remain a permanent mark, no matter how inconspicuous, where an incision has been made.

In some situations scars can heal unfavourably in certain people. Scars may become infected, stretched or thickened (*hypertrophic* or *keloid*) and may necessitate further treatment e.g. steroid injections or scar revision to improve the final cosmetic appearance. Even in someone who has never had a history of unfavourable scarring, the unexpected can occasionally happen and mar an otherwise good result.

Some areas of the body and some skin types are notorious for producing worse scars than others e.g. over the breastbone. Where an incision is sutured under tension there is a good chance that the scar will stretch, for example, in abdominoplasty (see pages 174–179).

If a ten-centimetre incision is made on the forearms of 100 individuals and sutured in exactly the same manner, the final outcome after two years would give a variety of results. At one end of the scale the scar would be almost invisible. At the other, a thickened, raised and red hypertrophic or keloid scar would result. This simple example also applies to more complex procedures; unfortunate healing such as this can thus give an unfavourable result to a procedure that has been otherwise expertly performed.

Pain and Discomfort

Following any surgical procedure the patient will experience a degree of pain and discomfort. Although research has given us an increased understanding of the mechanisms of pain and its perception by the human body, the best we can still do is to give appropriate medication in an attempt to alleviate or reduce pain, especially in the immediate postoperative period.

The degree and duration of postoperative pain will depend on the nature of the operation and the patient's pain threshold. Little can be done at present to alter an individual's pain threshold. The standard painkilling injections and tablets usually suffice to alleviate this unpleasant sensation to a tolerable degree.

It is therefore extremely difficult if not impossible to describe accurately to patients beforehand the degree and duration of their postoperative pain.

Bruising and Swelling

This is the body's natural response to injury. Every surgical procedure is followed by a period of bruising and swelling, depending on the nature and extent of the surgery.

In general, the more expert and adept a surgeon is, the less postoperative bruising and swelling will result. This is because an experienced and slick surgeon will perform an operation or procedure with the least amount of imparted trauma to the tissues.

The patient's response to trauma is also an important part of the equation. Some people bruise more easily than others and this can be caused by variations in the fragility of their blood vessels and the levels of blood coagulation (clotting) factors. Most elderly people have more fragile blood vessels than the young. Low levels of blood coagulation factors can run in families, even without obviously diagnosable bleeding disorders.

Although there has been much controversy about its effectiveness, many surgeons recommend a course of arnica tablets both before and after surgery to help reduce bruising and swelling and to enhance the healing process.

Bleeding and Haematoma

Sometimes bleeding can continue after the end of the operation or restart again several hours after completion of the operation. It can either track to the surface and manifest itself as localised bruising or collect in a space or pocket deep in the skin. Such a collection of blood is called a haematoma and if it becomes large enough (expanding haematoma) it will be necessary to remove or evacuate it through a further procedure.

In certain cosmetic procedures an expanding haematoma constitutes a surgical emergency in that, if it is not treated promptly, irreversible damage to the surrounding tissue can occur. The best example of this is an expanding haematoma developing under the skin flap following facelift surgery resulting in 'flap necrosis' or death of the skin.

Infection

Infection can occur after any surgical procedure. Most commonly the wound (incision site) is affected. If the infection progresses, the adjacent and surrounding tissues can become affected. This condition is known as *cellulitis*. Further progression of the infection may lead to formation of a localised deep pocket of pus or *abscess* formation.

Fortunately, infection in cosmetic surgery is not common and is easily treatable, usually with antibiotics, rest and local hygiene measures. Abscess formation must be more vigorously treated, often necessitating further surgical intervention in the form of a drainage procedure. Abscess formation is extremely rare but can occur following some cosmetic procedures, such as breast surgery, abdominoplasty and liposuction.

Sometimes chest infections occur after surgery, especially in smokers and patients with previous chest or breathing problems.

Finally it must be mentioned that MRSA (methicillin resistant staphylococcus aureus or 'superbug' as it is labelled by the press) is increasingly becoming the scourge of our hospitals. If an MRSA infection is diagnosed, it can be extremely difficult to treat. It is rare in previously healthy patients who only spend a short time in hospital, which is the usual situation in cosmetic surgery.

Deep Vein Thrombosis

This complication is rare in patients undergoing elective cosmetic surgery. Deep vein thrombosis (DVT) results when a blood clot develops in one or more deep veins in the calf. It is possible for the clot to become dislodged from its origin in the calf and be transported by the bloodstream to the lungs (pulmonary embolus) where it can have very serious consequences. Patients with a previous history of postoperative deep vein thrombosis should warn the surgeon and the anaesthetist before the operation.

Women taking oral contraceptives may run a slightly increased risk of developing a deep vein thrombosis after some operations. There is some controversy about the benefit of stopping oral contraceptives before surgery. Many medical practitioners hold the view that an equal or even greater risk is incurred from the possible complications of an unwanted pregnancy upon cessation of the pill. Nevertheless, it is thought wise to stop oral contraceptives prior to certain operations. Every patient is assessed on merit before surgery and the surgeon should advise each patient accordingly.

Nowadays the best equipped hospitals and clinics have equipment that massages the calves while the patient is under general anaesthetic. In addition, it is now standard practice for all patients to wear anti-embolism stockings during and after the operation.

The incidence of DVT is very much reduced if patients resume gentle activity soon after the operation. It is not a good idea to spend several days in bed after surgery if it is possible to get up and move about. This is not to say that patients should strenuously exercise soon after surgery, as this is likely to have a very deleterious effect.

Allergic Reactions to Drugs and Dressings

Various drugs are given during a hospital stay in the ward or injected during the course of a general anaesthetic. It is important to avoid being given any drug to which you might be allergic. You must report any known allergy especially to drugs, dressings and foods to the nursing staff on admission to hospital. Severe allergic responses have to be dealt with promptly and effectively to avoid serious consequences.

Blood Transfusion

Blood transfusion is seldom required in cosmetic surgery. All blood is carefully screened by the blood transfusion service for any infectious agent before it is released for use.

Drains

Sometimes small flexible tubes are used to enable collections of blood or other fluids to drain out from a wound. This reduces bruising and speeds recovery. They are removed a day or two after the operation. Modern drains are made of pliable plastic and remove easily without causing discomfort.

Problems with Urination or Urinary Tract Infection

Patients who are prone to urinary or kidney infections have an increased risk of this happening after surgery. This may be due to lying in one position for a prolonged period during the operation and its recovery, and also because drinking a lot of water is discouraged immediately before surgery.

The Preoperative Consultation

The results of cosmetic surgery can be very gratifying to both the patient and the surgeon. Before you have any treatment, a consultation with the surgeon should take place, involving a full discussion without any obligation. All your questions should be answered satisfactorily and you should be given time to think over what has been said and what has been proposed.

In an ideal world, cosmetic surgery should consist of two parties only: you and the surgeon. After all, it is the surgeon who has the task of determining your expectations, performing the operation or procedure, looking after you postoperatively and taking full responsibility for all postoperative problems, complications or unfavourable consequences.

Without doubt, the single most important stage in any cosmetic surgical procedure is the preoperative consultation. It is at this stage that all the necessary parameters are laid down. In addition, both you and the surgeon should form an amicable relationship based on honesty, integrity and trust. If such a relationship is not formed at this stage it is better in the long term for you to seek help elsewhere or for the surgeon to decline treatment because the likelihood of an outcome unsatisfactory to you is very much increased.

A consultation is essential because the surgeon also has to ask you about your past medical history in order to find out if there are any details that might influence an operation. When the surgeon knows more about you he is then in a better position to operate effectively and safely. The surgeon will normally communicate with your GP after the consultation, as long as you have given him permission to do so.

At the initial consultation the surgeon has a duty to decide if you have a problem that can be improved by an operation. Sometimes your feelings about what you look like are very different from what other people see. The best results in cosmetic surgery are obtained when the surgeon and the patient agree about the problem in the first instance. Then the surgeon has to ask himself whether there is an appropriate treatment that will improve it. It is obviously pointless to undertake a treatment that might not work or might even make things worse. In order to be successful, an operation has to be performed on the right person using the right technique.

Once the surgeon has decided that there is a treatment that will work, he should inform you fully about the operation and the postoperative course of events, such as when the stitches are removed and when you can expect to be 'presentable' again after the operation.

Cosmetic surgery is not invisible. But, by careful operative technique and the accurate positioning of the incisions, the scars can be almost invisible and only detectable on the closest examination. Patients on their part should realise that some skin heals better than others (see pages 37–38). This, of course, should be fully discussed in the initial consultation – as should *all* likely complications. The more you know about the operation because everything has been carefully explained to you, the more likely you are to be pleased with the result. This initial consultation can take up to an hour, in order for the surgeon to tell you enough about the operation for you to be able to make a valid decision. Most surgeons these days hand out printed information sheets that can be studied carefully later.

The initial consultation is a mutual process: both you and the surgeon will be trying to assess each other. You will be trying to decide whether to allow the surgeon to treat you. There are three criteria that are important in this assessment process:

1. Does the surgeon understand the problem? Did he make the appropriate responses when you explained the problem? Understanding the patient's problem is vital, because if the surgeon never quite empathised with the patient, a successful outcome would be a fluke. You need to consider whether the treatment proposed by the surgeon is actually what you are seeking and whether it is relevant to your problem.

2. Did the surgeon prove to you that he can do something about it successfully? At consultation, most surgeons show photographs of previous patients, which should give you a good idea of what the surgeon is likely to achieve. You should ensure that the photographs are relevant to your own case. If you are unconvinced by the photographs of the surgeon's previous patients, you should not go ahead.

3. Has anything put you off from wanting to be a patient of this particular surgeon? Sometimes the photographs reveal that the surgeon's and your ideas of what would be a successful result are radically different. Your judgment should not be solely determined by the reputation and qualifications of the surgeon. Not all surgeons are right for all patients and vice versa. To have a cosmetic operation performed by any particular surgeon is a very personal choice. It is important to establish a good rapport. If you are put off for any reason you should seek another surgeon.

The surgeon's job at the preoperative interview is simpler. There is only one criterion: whether he thinks you are going to be pleased if you have the proposed treatment. If the surgeon feels that there is a significant risk of disappointment then he would be unlikely to offer it.

Of course, you may decide not to go ahead after hearing all about the operation. The consultation will still have been very valuable and saved you a lot of stress and worry – and money! There should be no pressure to come to a decision at the consultation itself. On the contrary, difficult decisions, such as deciding whether to have an operation or not, must not be rushed.

Most surgeons will offer you several consultations, anticipating that you will often only think of important questions that you wish you had asked after you have given the matter a good deal of thought. Some patients may wish to book their surgery at the initial consultation in a wave of enthusiasm, only to regret it later. Commercial clinics and greedy surgeons have certainly put pressure on patients to decide quickly and have offered inducements to do so. This is extremely unprofessional practice.

The surgeon himself should of course carry out the initial consultation, the surgery and all the postoperative care, and should be available to you at all times during the treatment process.

Some surgeons use computer imaging to illustrate or emphasise possible results or outcomes of surgery. This technique may work well and be successful for some surgeons and patients. Neither of us adopt this practice routinely, because we are only too aware that it is not always possible to accurately match the final long-term postoperative appearance of a part of the body by simply editing features on a computer screen. The human body does not always comply with the before and after pictures illustrated by computer graphics for reasons already explained. We therefore urge extreme caution to all patients who have experienced a consultation where computer imaging was used – the result shown may not necessarily match the result achieved by surgery.

It is a sensible idea to see a number of surgeons before going ahead with an operation. This makes it much easier to assess individual surgeons against each other, and to decide which surgeon would be most appropriate for you.

Throughout this book we emphasise that the preoperative consultation is perhaps the most important part of the whole process of undergoing a cosmetic surgical procedure. The relationship between the patient and surgeon is of the utmost importance. No other adviser, so-called counsellor or any other party should interfere or be involved in the counselling stage. To make the point again: beware of establishments that offer the services of such people.

Preoperative Considerations

In order to get the best possible result for a particular patient it is extremely important to strive to attain the best possible conditions in which to operate. It is our opinion that the preoperative consultation is the most important part of the entire cosmetic procedure, and has been discussed in more detail in the previous section. This section deals with the physical and medical aspects of the fitness of a patient for surgery.

Because cosmetic surgery is entirely elective, it is of paramount importance for the surgeon to ensure that you are physically fit to withstand the operation safely and without undue risk. It would be extremely foolhardy for a surgeon to operate on any patient who has an increased risk of a serious medical complication following a procedure, which may endanger her well-being.

A carefully devised pre-consultation questionnaire is a useful tool to screen a patient from a purely medical perspective. This will usually give the surgeon all the information he requires in order to ascertain if you are physically fit for surgery, or if there are any factors that may preclude proceeding. Any grey areas can then be investigated in more detail.

In addition, the surgeon will go through his own, thorough screening routine to ensure that it is safe to operate on you. Some of the more important points to consider are as follows.

Your Current General Health

Any significant history of current problems with medical fitness will immediately alert the surgeon to take appropriate action and make an informed decision regarding proceeding with surgery. You should report any recently encountered symptoms, e.g. excessive thirst, frequency of passing urine, unexplained weight loss, as these may signify the onset of an illness that has previously been undiagnosed, such as diabetes.

Past Medical History

A detailed past medical history should help uncover any contraindications to proceeding with surgery or alert the surgeon to any possible postoperative problems e.g. previous postoperative deep vein thrombosis, or a history of heart or chest problems.

You should declare any past psychiatric history, with accurate details of any hospital admissions and medications prescribed. A past history of depression or anxiety can be very relevant to how you react to the stress of having an operation.

Current Medications

It is important to inform your surgeon of any oral medications you may be taking, in case they are likely to react with any medication likely to be given during an anaesthetic or at any time in hospital. Of particular importance is the oral contraceptive pill and hormone-replacement therapy, as in some situations it will be necessary to take extra steps to protect the patient against the possibility of postoperative deep vein thrombosis.

You should also declare any homeopathic, alternative or other medicines or preparations to the surgeon and anaesthetist before surgery. These too can interact with conventional medicines, especially anaesthetic drugs, which could have disastrous consequences. (See Appendix, page 231.)

Allergies

By the time a person reaches puberty, she should be aware of any allergies she may be suffering from, especially to conventional drugs. The commonest, most important and pertinent allergen in surgery is Penicillin. Obviously an allergy to any other drug or medication is also important, especially to a particular anaesthetic agent or post anaesthetic drug, but this is less common. All allergies should therefore be declared prior to surgery.

Family Medical History

Any significant family history of illness should be declared, especially a family history of anaesthetic problems. A condition known as Malignant Hyperthermia is a familial disorder, whereby the sufferer's metabolic rate is grossly enhanced when under a general anaesthetic leading to a grossly exaggerated and rapid rise in body temperature, which, if not promptly and expertly treated, can lead to the rapid demise of the patient. Thankfully, this condition is extremely rare.

You should declare any other disease or illness that you know runs in your family, no matter how insignificant you think it to be.

Bleeding/Clotting Disorders

Any bleeding tendency or abnormal clotting disorder in you or your family must be fully investigated before surgery. Prior to surgery, many patients complain of 'bruising easily'. This is usually a harmless disorder, often referred to as 'devil's pinch', and is not significant.

If you or your relatives have previously experienced deep vein thrombosis following surgery, you should be treated with the utmost care and given prophylactic preventative therapy prior to surgery.

An increasing number of patients are travelling long distances by air to undergo cosmetic surgery (see pages 34–35). There is an increasing number of fatalities from pulmonary embolus (see page 40) in patients who have recently stepped off a plane and gone straight into an operating theatre for surgery. Extreme caution should always be exercised in these circumstances.

Abnormal Healing/Scarring

A history of abnormal scarring or healing should prepare you and your surgeon for the possibility of an unfavourable result. Everything possible should be done in an attempt to minimise this complication e.g. your strict adherence to postoperative instructions, and measures for the prevention of infection. (See 'Risk Factors Common to All Operations', pages 36–41.)

Vitamins

The taking of vitamins is encouraged in order to enhance healing. The homeopathic preparation arnica is recommended by many surgeons as an aid to healing, although some scientific reports have cast doubt over its effectiveness.

Smoking

All patients are strongly encouraged to stop smoking. Smoking is not only a recognised health hazard in its own right, but is responsible for a number of postoperative problems and complications in patients who have a general anaesthetic for elective cosmetic surgery.

Chest infections

Heavy smokers are more likely to develop a chest infection postoperatively, particularly after major procedures such as abdominoplasty.

Impaired circulation

It is a known fact that heavy smokers are more liable to suffer the consequences of impaired circulation. This can lead to flap necrosis (loss of the skin resulting in noticeable scars) e.g. following a facelift or abdominoplasty. The rate of healing will also be affected. In addition, a smokers cough immediately following facelift surgery can easily precipitate a haemorrhage and an expanding haematoma (see page 39).

Excessive Alcohol Intake

Excessive alcohol intake will impair liver function and therefore the production of the essential clotting factors in the blood. This can sometimes cause a problem if the clotting time is increased after the operation. This can in turn lead to excessive postoperative bleeding with the increased likelihood of developing a postoperative haematoma (see page 39).

Aspirin, a common drug taken for a variety of reasons, has a similar effect on bleeding, and should be avoided for two weeks prior to elective surgery if at all possible.

Anaesthetic Reactions

This has already been mentioned above (see page 47). Individual patients react differently to a general anaesthetic. Some suffer excessive vomiting, some find it difficult to wake up afterwards, some wake up very tearful, but luckily most get no side effects at all.

In many cases you will be aware of a particular reaction you have to an anaesthetic agent from previous experience. Any untoward reaction to an anaesthetic agent must be dealt with promptly and, thankfully, serious complications are rare. Any known anaesthetic reaction must therefore be declared prior to surgery.

Most local anaesthetics contain adrenaline. The function of the adrenaline is to cause vasoconstriction (narrowing of the local blood vessels) thereby reducing bleeding at the operation site. This makes it a lot easier for the surgeon to operate.

In the main, allergies to local anaesthetics are extremely rare. However, some people can occasionally develop an unpleasant feeling immediately following the injection of a local anaesthetic, which is attributable to the adrenaline. This reaction is usually short lived.

Abstinence from Food and Drink

Every patient undergoing a general anaesthetic must abstain from food and drink for several hours beforehand. This is to ensure that the stomach is empty in order to prevent the inhalation of vomit during the administration and duration of the anaesthetic. Each patient will be advised accordingly.

Urinary Problems

Urinary tract infections are a common postoperative complication, especially in patients who are prone to them (see page 41).

Employment and Social History

One of the commonest questions patients ask after surgery is, 'When can I go back to work?' The surgeon will need to know what your work commitments and circumstances entail in order to answer this question accurately. Depending on the scale of the procedure you are considering, you may need to arrange to have some considerable time off work. Only you will know if this is feasible. Your relationship with your work colleagues – whether you get on well with them or not, whether they know about and are sympathetic towards your having surgery – can also have an important bearing on how successfully you view the result.

Ideally you will have a loyal and supportive partner or close friend who will help you through the inevitable stress of having surgery and coping with the immediate effects. Often the result of surgery initially is quite disappointing. At first the patient just sees the effect of an injury: bruising, swelling, scars and stitches. It is only later that the beneficial effects of the operation become apparent. It is very helpful to have personal support through these early stages after an operation.

The second best situation is to be left alone to recover quietly without having to look after anyone else except yourself. The worst situation is to live with a partner who is antagonistic to the whole idea of the operation. Every little bruise could be the focus of an 'I told you so' type of remark, and an operation that would have been a success with a supportive partner can be turned into a failure.

It is a good idea for a husband and wife to attend the preoperative consultation together if possible, so that the events in the postoperative phase and all the complications and risks can be explained to them both at the same time. This is particularly pertinent to breast surgery and skin resurfacing procedures of the face.

Your Hopes and Expectations

One of the most important questions the surgeon should ask you is, 'What are you trying to achieve?' He then has to compare your answer to what you are actually likely to get. If you are hoping for rather more than the procedure is generally capable of achieving, then disappointment is very likely.

The ideal patients for cosmetic surgery are physically healthy, emotionally sound and want what the operation can usually provide. A supportive home and work environment also make a big difference.

Postoperative Concerns

The Immediate Phase

Most patients are understandably concerned about the events immediately after their surgical procedure.

Many who undergo cosmetic surgery for the first time in their life will probably not have experienced being in a hospital or a clinic environment before. This, together with concerns about postoperative pain, discomfort, bruising and swelling, will leave most patients in turmoil and in need of reassurance and support.

In our experience, the vast majority of patients usually cope extremely well and prospective patients need not be unduly concerned or worried about the after effects of their surgery.

Pain and discomfort are inevitable after most operations (see page 38). Those with a known low pain threshold are invariably more concerned. The fear of the unknown adds to their anxiety. Thankfully, the available medication for pain relief quickly alleviates their anxieties in the majority of cases.

For most patients, cosmetic surgery is a private matter and they don't want the world to know about it. Unfortunately, the telltale signs of surgery are pretty obvious for a few days. Operations on the face, nose and eyelids cause swelling and bruises that are initially hard to disguise. Many patients will attempt to hide away for a few days until the signs of recent surgery have disappeared.

Many patients tell their friends and family white lies to explain their appearance, suggesting that bruises and swelling have been caused by an accident. It is even possible to explain away a nasal splint after rhinoplasty. We do not, however, condone this. We feel it is much better for a patient to be honest about their surgery, and therefore enlist the help and support of their friends rather than continue in the deception. Obviously not *everyone* needs to know. A lot of patients will need a sick certificate to facilitate time off work after the operation. This is a legal document, and has to be accurate. It doesn't have to be *precisely* accurate though, and we often put, 'due to the effects of recent surgery' without saying exactly what that surgery was for.

Although, in our experience, the vast majority of patients are entirely satisfied with the results of their surgery and gladly accept their new appearance, we are met with the occasional surprise. It is not unknown for a patient to become very distressed and reject their new image when viewing the results for the first time. For example, this can occur as an initial reaction at the 'grand-unveiling' stage when the splint is taken off a nose following rhinoplasty.

Mercifully this reaction is usually short lived, and the patient quickly embraces their new image. Whether this occurs as a result of a panic attack, or some underlying psychological phenomenon, is hard to ascertain. Luckily, such reactions are very rare but they are nevertheless disconcerting for the patient and surgeon alike.

Long-Term Phase

Several cosmetic procedures take weeks or even months to settle fully before the final resting phase is established. Common examples of this are rhinoplasty, liposuction, breast reduction and abdominoplasty.

Long-term swelling and discomfort do occasionally occur with some procedures and this adds to patient anxiety. Scarring is also a worry for some, especially if the scar is not settling down very well and still looks unsightly after some time.

Scars go through three stages after surgery. Initially they are generally nice and neat, but after a few months they become red and raised, and then settle down, hopefully into thin white lines, the whole process taking up to a year or so. Massaging with skin cream helps scars to settle. In those patients who have a tendency to form lumpy scars, surgical tape applied at night can minimise the problem. If a scar really does become a problem, injections of steroid into the scar are very effective at shrinking it. If steroid injections do not have an adequate beneficial effect, then scar revision can be considered (see 'Improving Unsightly Scars', pages 196–199). However, there isn't much point in doing a scar revision before it is mature because there is still a chance that it will settle down.

Some generally successful operations do have specific problems, such as breasts becoming hard with breast implants (see pages 148–149), or polly beak deformity (see page 134) after rhinoplasty. You will naturally seek reassurance from your surgeon, who will do his best to explain the problem and advise accordingly.

Self image

Many people prefer not to tell anyone if they are having cosmetic surgery. They are concerned that their friends or peers will laugh at them, or worse, deride them for undergoing what they think is a trivial and frivolous procedure. Some people may have been teased or bullied by their peers for their original blemish. They may be very worried about having their surgical 'correction' of this 'defect' found out, because it may only exacerbate that former teasing, once that 'correction' is noticed.

In reality, the average onlooker (including close friends and relatives), will rarely notice an alteration in someone's appearance unless it is pretty dramatic. This is purely because the human brain so quickly forgets what went before, without reference to some previous photograph image.

Consider the typical magazine competition puzzle 'Spot the Difference'. Two seemingly identical drawings or pictures, placed next to each other, have a number of differences. With the two pictures alongside, one can eventually spot the differences. Likewise, only when comparing before-and-after photographs of a patient, will the difference in appearance become obvious.

However, when a patient first meets a friend or acquaintance after their operation, this friend is unlikely to have a preoperative photograph to hand to compare it with. It is unlikely that they will, specifically, notice any difference. Some observers do sometimes suspect that there is a difference, but they cannot put their finger on exactly what the difference is.

In the main, patients need not be apprehensive about undergoing surgery on this purely social level. Very few, if any, of their closest friends will notice. To make it even harder to 'spot the difference' we advise patients to make some other, more conspicuous alteration to their appearance, such as a change of hairstyle or hair-colour. People may well then say, 'Your new hairstyle really suits you, it makes you look so much younger,' without even suspecting a facelift!

Really successful cosmetic surgery should produce a dramatic improvement in appearance, so that it boosts your confidence, while simultaneously being virtually unnoticeable. Cosmetic surgeons need to be artists as well as technicians.

It is possible to get slightly hooked on cosmetic surgery; it is very moreish after all! Some patients have too many operations and do eventually get to look slightly odd – we've all seen the photos in the celebrity magazines. Those more flamboyant types, such as young women who want the largest possible breast implants or fullest possible lips tend to attract adverse criticism from sections of the public and media. Any ethical and responsible surgeon should warn his patient when this limit is approaching, and advise her accordingly.

The Causes of Disappointment

Although cosmetic surgery is generally very successful, the best surgeon in the world will occasionally have patients who are bitterly disappointed with their treatment. This disappointment may occur in any of the three following stages:

1. The counselling/consultation stage. The surgeon and patient did not communicate properly so the patient did not get the result she was expecting.

2. During the operation. Perhaps a medical problem caused the result to be poor, or the standard of the surgery was simply not good enough. Surgeons are usually blamed if there are problems, but there are many factors that can affect surgery that are not under the surgeon's control, however skilled and experienced he or she may be.

3. After the operation. Some sort of complication perhaps, or the patient is frustrated at the length of time it takes to recover or come to terms with the change in appearance. Perhaps the worst scenario occurs when the final result is below the standard that would normally be expected from the procedure.

Counselling and Consultation

Communication by talking is actually a very difficult skill. Almost everyone misses the point or misunderstands when they talk to other people at some time. Sometimes two people click as soon as they meet, but usually one needs to know someone very well indeed in order never to misunderstand them.

Spoken words conjure up images in the brain of the listener that can be totally different from those that were being described by the speaker. Words such as 'small' or 'better' can change their meaning entirely as they pass between the two. Comfortable, stress-free conditions and sufficient time can make all the difference to the outcome of an interview.

Many patients are nervous and embarrassed when they first meet a surgeon, which can be a barrier to effective communication. The surgeon should be able to relax the patient by a calm and unhurried approach. However good a surgeon is at operating, there is more to the job than that. The surgeon needs to have a sympathetic manner and make it easy for patients to talk about their problems.

If, after a consultation, you feel that you have not been able to say all you wanted to say, or felt that you have been misunderstood, you would be best advised to seek another consultation, possibly even see another surgeon, before you decide whether to have the operation.

At the initial consultation, the surgeon will be carefully evaluating your response to his questions and will be trying to decide exactly what you are hoping to get out of the operation. The result that you expect has to match closely the result that the surgeon is likely to achieve. If you are expecting something that is beyond the prowess of the surgeon, or is not a normal result of the operation itself, then disappointment is the likely outcome.

A few patients are disappointed with an operation that has been performed perfectly, and where any objective observer would think there has been an excellent result. The problem here is that there has been a failure of communication between the patient and the surgeon, and a mismatch between patient expectation and what has been achievable.

Photographs of the surgeon's previous patients are a great help because they can give a good impression of what the operation can do for you and the surgeon can observe your response. If you feel that the results shown in the photographs are disappointing, then the surgeon should discuss with you whether your expectations are unreasonably high. You should be advised not to proceed. If you form the view in consultation with the surgeon that the surgeon's results will not please you then it would be foolish to go any further.

Occasionally expectations can change during the course of the treatment. Whereas at the initial consultation you may have felt that any improvement would be a satisfactory result, afterwards you may be disappointed that the result is not more dramatic.

The surgeon should be forthcoming to you about the negative side of the operation, such as scarring or the possibility of the result changing with time. Any patient is likely to be disappointed if she did not know that an inevitable result of her operation would be significant scarring, for example. It is essential that you listen carefully to any description of negative effects, and take them seriously.

All cosmetic surgeons occasionally see patients who they feel will not be happy afterwards, for any number of reasons. Patient selection – that is, only agreeing to operate on candidates who have realistic expectations and are likely to be pleased with the results – is an important part of any surgeon's responsibility.

Cosmetic surgery counsellors

An increasing number of establishments advertise cosmetic surgery in the media. Many of these are run by non-medically qualified persons, who are not bound by medical ethics. They pursue clever marketing methods, including hard-sell tactics, to entice prospective patients to attend their establishment.

In addition, many employ the services of so called 'counsellors'. These counsellors come from various backgrounds, from nursing to sales. These persons are specifically trained to sell the operation to every patient they see. They are usually remunerated on a commission-only basis, meaning that they only get paid if the prospective patient elects to have treatment. The implications of this should be obvious to everyone concerned.

It is our recommendation and opinion that any patient who wishes to undergo cosmetic surgery only be counselled by the operating surgeon and NOT by any other party. Every patient is unique and has specific requirements and expectations. How can an independent person who has absolutely no previous operating experience advise patients about an operation when even two experienced surgeons may not necessarily agree on a treatment plan or achieve the same result?

In clinics where several surgeons are employed, patients should ensure that they are only operated on by the surgeon who counselled them initially, provided they were happy with him in the first place.

In the case where a third party or so-called 'counsellor' is involved, the usual reason for disappointment is due to the patient being misled in some way. Either the result was not as promised or the nature of the operation, complications and sequelae were not adequately explained or discussed.

Statistics clearly show that nearly all causes of disappointment are due to poor patient selection and inadequate or inappropriate preoperative counselling. This is far more likely to occur if another party is involved in the surgeon-patient relationship.

During the Operation

There is no substitute for skill and experience, and a genuine interest in cosmetic surgery on the part of the surgeon. Although cosmetic surgeons are drawn from a number of different specialities, all are motivated by how their patients will look after the operation. Nevertheless, all surgeons (and not just cosmetic surgeons) sometimes produce results that are not up to their usual standard. Sometimes this is a minor problem, such as a misplaced suture slightly distorting the edge of a wound. Or, it could be a more significant error, such as the removal of too much skin in trying to correct a crease. Overall, such consequences of surgery are unusual.

Much more likely is the situation where something happens that is outside the surgeon's control, such as an allergic drug reaction or where a patient has a bleeding tendency that was unsuspected before the operation. This can make the achievement of an optimum result very difficult indeed. Although technical perfection is the aim during the operation it is not always possible and the preoperative counselling of the patient should take this into account.

Nowadays anaesthesia is not nearly as risky or problematic as it used to be, and a healthy patient has little to fear from a routine anaesthetic.

After the Operation

A fully informed patient should know what to expect after their surgery, and be better able to cope with minor discomfort and the appearance of the new wounds. Bruising, swelling and soreness are a feature of most operations and this can be a shock to some patients, even though they knew about it in advance. Other patients may be disappointed that full recovery can take some time after the operation.

Postoperative complications can occur as in all surgery. Especially important are the risks of infection and bleeding (see pages 39–40), both of which can mar an otherwise good result. Some areas of the body and some patients scar badly however neatly and expertly the surgeon treats them (see pages 37–38).

If the result of a cosmetic operation is disappointing because of some technical problem, it is nearly always possible to correct the defect and produce a successful outcome by further revision surgery.

In those few unfortunate cases where there is a good technical result but where the patient is dissatisfied, further surgery is unlikely to be very effective and both surgeon and patient may come to regret the decision to operate in the first place.

Anaesthesia

Many patients are more worried about having a general anaesthetic than undergoing their operation. You may be concerned that something could happen which might mean you won't wake up again, or that you will lose control and behave in an undignified way while asleep. The motto of the Association of Anaesthetists is 'Safety in sleep'. Nowadays anaesthetics are very safe, and rapidly induced and reversed. Once asleep, you are in the hands of a trained specialist and are carefully monitored throughout the entire procedure.

The type of anaesthetic that is used depends on the nature and extent of the operation, the wishes of the patient and the preference of the surgeon. Sometimes factors in your medical history or previous experience of anaesthetics influence the decision.

Essentially there are three types of anaesthetic: local, regional and general.

Local Anaesthetic

The part of the body to be operated on is numbed by injecting a local anaesthetic agent directly into the tissue. There is usually an initial brief stinging sensation whilst the anaesthetic is being administered, after which the area will become totally numb. You will be aware of what is going on around you but will not experience any unpleasant sensation such as pain or discomfort.

It is usual to give oral sedatives prior to injection of local anaesthetic for very nervous patients who have 'needle phobia'. For some procedures heavy sedation is combined with local anaesthetic and this is known as a 'twilight anaesthetic'. Some surgeons favour a twilight anaesthetic for certain procedures, such as facelifts.

In most situations the local anaesthetic is mixed with adrenaline to prolong the effect of the anaesthetic as well as reduce bleeding in the area injected (the adrenaline narrows the blood vessels in the injected area).

Regional Anaesthetic

Using this technique a specific area of the body is numbed. Regional anaesthesia is increasingly used to avoid the possible side effects of a general anaesthetic. The following types of regional anaesthesia are commonly used.

Nerve Block

Some procedures are performed using a technique known as a nerve block. This technique requires a detailed knowledge of the anatomy of the nerve supply to the area to be operated on. Local anaesthetic is injected into the tissue immediately in the vicinity of the targeted nerve trunk. The local anaesthetic is absorbed into the nerve sheath and temporarily interrupts conduction of nerve impulses thereby numbing the entire area, which is supplied by the nerve.

In cosmetic surgery, nerve block is most commonly used for procedures on the face. The entire face can be numbed with a few strategically sited injections. More commonly, specific parts of the face are numbed so that a procedure can be performed without pain e.g. on the lips and nose.

Spinal anaesthetic

This technique involves the injection of local anaesthetic into the fluid that surrounds the nerves in the lower part of the spine. It is therefore used for procedures below the waist and in the pelvic area. You are completely numb from the waist down for a few hours.

Epidural anaesthetic

This is a similar technique to a spinal anaesthetic. A narrow plastic tube is inserted and left in position near the nerves in the lower part of the spine. Repeated doses of local anaesthetic can be administered through this tube without further injections to prolong the duration and effect.

General Anaesthetic

With a general anaesthetic you are put to sleep and will be completely unaware of what is going on. When the operation is completed the anaesthetic is reversed and you wake up again.

Recent years have seen the development of new, safer anaesthetic drugs, and sophisticated, computerised monitoring equipment. Nowadays general anaesthetics are very safe and you need not be apprehensive or fearful of being put to sleep. Millions of anaesthetics are successfully performed throughout the world every year.

Before the operation
Patients who smoke should give up or cut down as much as possible in the weeks before (see page 48–49). It is also recommended to drink less alcohol than usual, especially in average or heavy drinkers (see page 49). If you get a cough, cold or some other illness shortly before the date of admission you should inform the clinic, as it might be sensible to postpone the operation.

Patients are usually asked to arrive some time before the operation is due to allow time for the anaesthetist to examine them and ask questions that are relevant to the giving of an anaesthetic. If you are taking tablets or any medication you should bring them with you to the clinic. Some medical treatments can interfere with anaesthetics and cause problems (see page 47). The anaesthetist will be particularly interested in previous anaesthetics that you have had and whether there were any problems (see pages 47 and 49). The anaesthetist may arrange for blood tests and urine tests to be done.

Anaesthetics can induce vomiting, so it is very important that the stomach is empty when the operation begins. You are not allowed to eat or drink for some hours before an operation. Sometimes a premedication – in the form of a sedative tablet or injection – is given about an hour before the operation. You are asked to change into an operating gown because ordinary clothes cannot be worn in the theatre.

In the anaesthetic room
You are brought to the anaesthetic room, which is usually a side room leading into the operating theatre. A careful check is made to ensure that no mistakes of identification have occurred and that the consent form for the operation has been signed. Leads (wires) are routinely stuck to various parts of the body using small adhesive plates. These wires are then connected to sophisticated monitors so that your vital signs can be carefully checked throughout the operation.

The anaesthetist inserts a thin plastic tube (cannula) into a vein, usually in the back of your hand. A plastic tube connects the cannula to a bag of sterile fluid. This is known as an intravenous infusion set. Fluid can therefore be run into your vein. In addition, anaesthetic drugs can be injected through this system directly into the vein.

The anaesthetist injects a drug that makes you rapidly go to sleep. This stage is known as the 'induction of anaesthesia'. Other drugs can then be given to prolong the anaesthetic. A plastic tube is put through your mouth into the windpipe to provide you with oxygen and anaesthetic gas during the procedure.

During the operation

You are then taken into the operating theatre and the operation begins. To maintain this unconscious state a mixture of oxygen and anaesthetic gases are given to you to breathe. This phase of anaesthesia is known as 'maintenance of anaesthesia' and you will not be aware of what is going on; you will be completely unconscious.

The anaesthetist keeps a very close watch and gives further drugs as necessary. It is sometimes necessary to give muscle-relaxing drugs in order to relax the body's natural muscle tone, still present during sleep, to enable the surgeon to perform the operation under the best possible conditions.

When a muscle relaxant is used, the muscles responsible for breathing are effectively paralysed as well, and the anaesthetist has to control the patient's breathing with a 'ventilator', a machine that blows oxygen and anaesthetic into the lungs via the tube in the windpipe.

Throughout the duration of the anaesthetic your condition is constantly monitored using sophisticated machinery to measure your vital signs. The parameters are the rate and electrical activity of the heart, blood pressure and the amount of oxygen in the blood.

When the operation has finished the anaesthetic gases are stopped and a drug is given to reverse the muscle relaxation so that you can breathe by yourself. You are then transferred to the recovery room and allowed to wake up fully. Often painkillers and drugs to control nausea are given at this time. When you have sufficiently recovered you are taken back to the ward and can then sleep off the rest of the anaesthetic.

After the operation

You may feel a bit groggy for a while, depending on the length of the operation, and often a bit sick. Nowadays recovery from a modern anaesthetic is much quicker than it used to be, and the after effects are much less severe. Strong drugs are available to deal with pain and nausea.

If you leave the clinic soon after the operation you may still be slightly under the influence of the anaesthetic. Legally, you must not drive or operate machinery until at least 24 hours after you have come round.

Complications

Apart from nausea and vomiting, complications are rare after a routine general anaesthetic. There is, however, a small risk of developing a chest infection (see pages 39–40) or deep vein thrombosis in the calves (see page 40). Allergies to anaesthetic drugs are rare, and the anaesthetist will be ready to deal with any untoward events that may occur.

The Routine Admission to a Clinic

Most patients are asked to attend the clinic on the day of the operation or sometimes the night before. Most clinics will require you to be admitted quite early in the day, some time before the operation, so that blood tests can be done and the results obtained. This also gives the surgeon and anaesthetist a chance to see you and answer any last minute questions you may have.

If you are travelling by car it is important that the driver is familiar with the route and adequate time has been allowed for difficulties in finding the clinic and any possible delays. A good safety margin in the timing of the journey by public transport is essential to allow you to arrive at the clinic in good time without being stressed and hurried. Having any sort of surgery is stressful enough in itself.

If you are driving yourself, you should make sure that your return journey is not within 24 hours of the anaesthetic. Soon after the operation it is strongly advised that someone else should take the stress of driving for you. It is amazing how many patients ignore this advice and still attempt to drive themselves home. But the rule is, 'Do not drive home after any surgical procedure'.

Once at the clinic, you will go through the admission procedure, which is usually carried out by the nurses. They will carefully fill out medical history forms and will attach an identity bracelet to your wrist. They will familiarise you with the clinic facilities and will be generally knowledgeable and forthcoming about your surgery and recovery. Blood and urine may be taken for routine tests. The nurses and the anaesthetist will make sure that you have not had anything to eat or drink for some hours before the operation if a general anaesthetic is going to be used.

You will be asked to change out of your ordinary clothes and put on an operation gown. It is never a good idea to bring valuables to a clinic, but rings and watches etc. that will have to be removed before the operation should be entrusted to the nurses for safekeeping. Jewellery that cannot be removed is generally taped over with surgical strapping. This is done to prevent burns that may be caused by the operation: if a metal object in contact with the skin touches part of the operating table it can act as a conduit for the electric current that is used by the surgeon to stop bleeding.

The anaesthetist will attach a device to a finger during the operation that measures the oxygen level in your blood. This gadget won't work very well in the presence of nail varnish, so nail varnish needs to be removed before the operation. It is customary to remove all other make-up as well. You should bring to the clinic enough toiletries to last you for your expected stay.

An essential part of the admission procedure is to gain legal consent for the operation. The surgeon usually does this personally. Often you are also asked to sign information sheets about the operation to ensure that you have given fully informed consent.

The anaesthetist will pay you a visit and ask a series of questions about previous anaesthetics and illnesses relevant to the anaesthetic (see 'Anaesthesia', pages 60–63). Further medical tests may be arranged. If necessary the anaesthetist will order a sedative drug to be given to you an hour or so before the start of the operation. You will usually be given some idea of the expected start time of your operation, but this can only be a guide, and delays during operating lists are frequent.

Shortly before the operation, porters or nurses will conduct you to the anaesthetic room where you will be given an anaesthetic. The first part of this will involve the anaesthetist's assistant, who will check your identity, make sure you have signed the consent form and that all the other paperwork is in order. Monitoring equipment such as ECG electrodes (which allow the anaesthetist to see the state of the heart at all times) and blood oxygen sensors are attached. These are all designed to make the anaesthetic safer.

Next, a needle will be inserted into a convenient vein, usually on the back of your non-dominant hand (i.e. the hand you do not write with). This is the only part of the induction of the anaesthetic that is uncomfortable, and it is only for a moment. The anaesthetist will then begin to inject a number of drugs using this needle. The cocktail of drugs will often include painkillers, sedatives, antibiotics and drugs to reduce nausea and vomiting afterwards. Then the anaesthetist will inject the anaesthetic itself. Modern induction agents, as they are called, act very rapidly and you will go to sleep in a matter of seconds. The anaesthetist will then pass a tube down your throat into the windpipe, so that anaesthetic gas can be delivered from the anaesthetic machine, which keeps you asleep during the operation. (See 'Anaesthesia', pages 60–63, for more detailed information about anaesthetics.)

When you are stable under anaesthetic you are then wheeled into the operating theatre, and carefully transferred to the operating table. The surgeon will check your positioning on the table.

Sterile surgical drapes are then applied around the operation site, to allow access to the site while providing a sterile barrier to prevent micro-organisms gaining access to the open wound. The skin of the operation site will be washed with a preparation that kills bacteria. Once the surgeon and the assistants have carefully sterilised their hands, they put on surgical gowns and gloves and the operation begins. Many procedures start with the surgeon injecting local anaesthetic and adrenaline. This reduces the bleeding, makes the operation easier to perform and reduces postoperative pain.

At the end of the operation the surgeon will carefully dress the wound. The anaesthetist will then switch off the anaesthetic gases and inject a further cocktail of drugs to help recovery. You will be transferred from the operating table onto a trolley and wheeled into the recovery room.

When you come round from the anaesthetic you will be in the recovery room, but you are unlikely to remember this. Most patients only remember waking up back in their bed in the ward. Immediately after the operation the nurses will make frequent checks on you and will be ready to give the treatment ordered by the anaesthetist to reduce pain and nausea. You may have a drip running into an arm vein so that you can receive some fluid while you are unable to drink. The drip is removed when you feel better and start to drink again.

Recovery after most cosmetic operations is really quite rapid. Many patients are fit to go home – to rest – later on the same day or the morning afterwards. Postoperative instructions should be followed as closely as possible because they are designed to prevent complications and ensure the best healing.

You are usually given a telephone number to call in case of any problems and an outpatient appointment to see the surgeon in a few days. The immediate effect of a cosmetic operation tends to be swelling and bruising and the improvement in your appearance may take some time to become apparent.

It is absolutely essential that you keep your follow-up appointments. If for any reason you cannot keep an appointment, it is important to inform the clinic or surgeon and arrange an alternative one. It is especially important to attend any long-term follow-up appointments as some procedures take a while to settle before the final result is achieved.

Is Cosmetic Surgery *Really* for You?

Not every person who attends a consultation with the aim of undergoing cosmetic surgery will be a suitable candidate for that surgery. We have already emphasised the importance of the preoperative consultation with your surgeon. This is a mutual process. While you are, of course, the paying customer, and thus need to be entirely happy with the surgeon and his skills, it is also down to the surgeon to assess your suitability and decide whether to accept you for treatment or not.

The surgeon may flatly refuse treatment for reasons discussed below. On some occasions the surgeon may refer you to a colleague for a second opinion. If there is any doubt about your psychological status the surgeon may refer you for a psychiatric opinion. Mercifully, the vast majority of patients who present for cosmetic surgery are entirely suitable, and fulfill all the basic criteria necessary to achieve a favourable result. You need to:

- be physically fit
- have an easily visible blemish or deformity that is readily amenable to treatment
- be self-motivated
- have realistic expectations
- fully understand the nature of the procedure, the likely result and the possible postoperative complications and sequelae.

If an unsuitable patient is treated this will invariably end in disappointment for both the patient and her surgeon. Certain traits and characteristics may increase the risk of your dissatisfaction with surgery. It is the professional obligation of any ethical surgeon to screen prospective patients carefully. You can also ask yourself the following questions:

Are Your Expectations Realistic?

Are you asking your surgeon to make you look like a model whose picture you have torn out of a magazine? Are you expecting a complete and utter transformation? When you look at the photographic portfolio of your prospective surgeon's work, if you are dissatisfied with or critical of every single photograph, this is a sure sign that the results you are seeking may be unachievable. If you are a perfectionist in life generally, satisfaction with any surgical result is highly unlikely. Remember, the surgeon can only work with the 'raw materials' before him. Good cosmetic surgery should result in an improvement, while you still remain demonstrably 'you'.

Do You Like the Surgeon and His Staff?

Undergoing any cosmetic surgery is a deeply personal and intimate business. You need to develop a comfortable and trusting rapport with your surgeon and his staff, the people who will be looking after you throughout all stages of your treatment. Any antagonism is only likely to increase the likelihood of dissatisfaction with your treatment. In order for the clinic to give you the best possible treatment, it is important that you keep appointments and listen to any advice you are given. The surgeon's decision to offer you treatment is based on psychological factors as much as physical ones. The nature of your interactions with the clinic staff will be one indicator of your suitability for surgery.

Have You Had a Recent Relationship Break Up?

This set of circumstances may not necessarily preclude you from being suitable for cosmetic surgery. After all, getting that nose job you've always dreamed of might be a way of boosting your confidence again and making a fresh start. However, you should be extremely wary about seeking surgery when you are in an emotionally vulnerable state. This could lead you to have unrealistic expectations. The results of your cosmetic surgery are not going to prevent any relationship break-ups in the future.

Are You Being Motivated or Pressured by a Partner?

This scenario will invariably lead to problems for you. It is extremely important that you are honest with yourself and your surgeon about this matter. Pressure from a partner or spouse can lead to you having multiple procedures. You may be exposing yourself to further criticism if this partner is not pleased with the results of your surgery. If you are agreeing to have this surgery in an attempt to save a relationship, if and when that relationship eventually breaks down, you will probably discover that you are dissatisfied with the surgery and will not think it has been worthwhile.

Is Your 'Deformity' Imaginary or Exaggerated?

As we have stated before, the most successful surgery usually occurs when both the surgeon and patient have similar perceptions of the 'deformity' to be corrected. And of course, everyone is more self-conscious about an apparent imperfection than third parties will be. If however, you have got to a state where the tiniest blemish has become an overwhelming obstacle, or where you perceive a feature negatively that other observers can't even see, this is a strong indicator that you will still not actually be happy with the results of your surgery either.

Do You Have a History of Mental or Psychiatric Illness?

Again, a 'yes' answer to this question may not automatically exclude you from having cosmetic surgery. After all, many people will suffer a bout of mild to moderate depression at some point in their lives, perhaps after a bereavement or divorce. However, we strongly recommend that such times are not ideal moments to undergo cosmetic surgery. You will be emotionally vulnerable, and may be hoping that surgery will pull you out of your depression. A depressed mental state will predispose you to reacting negatively to the results of your surgery.

In our opinion, patients with any personality disorder or long psychiatric history (particularly if severe enough to warrant inpatient care) should never be operated on without the prior authorisation and full co-operation of their psychiatrist or GP. Failure to observe this rule will inevitably lead to serious problems.

Do You Need Numerous Consultations?

We fully encourage all patients to come back for a second consultation if they have any further queries. Indeed the Healthcare Commission insist that patients should be encouraged to do this routinely in order to ensure that they have been properly counselled and fully aware of the procedure prior to making an informed consent to proceed. Any professional and responsible surgeon will be only too glad to answer your questions and keep you fully informed.

However, if you find yourself asking for your third, fourth or fifth consultation, this is a strong indicator that you are not yourself sure about having the surgery, and you should not proceed further. If you have already shopped around several other surgeons, and cannot find any that you are happy with, this could well mean that your expectations are unrealistically high.

Do You Know What You Want?

Are you quite clear in your own mind about what you want? Are you able to communicate this to the surgeon? If you are very vague about what you are hoping for, the surgeon may not be able to understand what you really want.

Have You Already Been Refused Treatment Elsewhere?

If another cosmetic surgeon has already refused you surgery, for whatever reason, he probably had very good cause. Prospective patients may well not reveal this to any other surgeons for fear of getting refused again. However, if you find a surgeon who overlooks this previous obstacle, you must ask yourself very carefully if you trust him, and whether you are exposing yourself to a higher level of risk.

How Do You Expect to be Treated?

With respect, courtesy, professionalism and expert individual care, of course! Undergoing cosmetic surgery can be a huge decision, and you don't want to feel that you are on a conveyor belt. On the other hand do you think that you are somehow a special case, a VIP? Are you expecting five-star Hollywood treatment? Do you have some impossible demand to place on your surgeon, such as a need to be looking flawless at a wedding one week after your surgery? If you answer yes to any of these questions it is highly unlikely that you will be satisfied with your surgery, no matter how well it is performed.

PART TWO
THE PROCEDURES

Part One of this book should have helped you to weigh up all the broader factors involved in deciding whether to have cosmetic surgery. Now we move on to the procedures themselves. This part of the book deals specifically with all the cosmetic surgical and non-surgical procedures that are commonly performed today; the likely, specific postoperative course of events and the possible complications. We have tried to avoid complex medical jargon, but the glossary at the end of the book should explain any medical terms with which you may not be familiar.

It is important to realise at the outset that cosmetic surgery follows the same rules as any other branch of surgery. Any operation is a physical assault on the human body, which can result in complications. Before reading about a particular procedure it is important to read 'Risk Factors Common to All Operations', beforehand, in order to gain a more comprehensive understanding of what may be involved.

Despite reading about a particular procedure, it will not give you all the information you require. As every prospective patient is unique, a consultation with the operating surgeon is essential in order to make an informed decision to proceed.

Cosmetic Surgery to the Face

FACELIFT

The History of the Facelift

The first facelift was performed over 100 years ago. It was a relatively simple operation by today's standards. A small piece of skin was removed from the scalp above the ear and the facial skin was pulled up to close the wound. The result was roughly similar to the effect of pulling the hair up into a ponytail. Unfortunately, in most patients the scar stretched after a few months and the skin came down again. It worked better in some patients whose soft skin pulled up easily.

It was soon discovered, however, that if the front edge of the wound was undermined (lifted or dissected) so that the skin of the temporal region was lifted away from its base, this skin could be moved more readily backwards and upwards. During the healing phase after the operation this skin would reattach, but at a higher point than before. This enabled the pull from the operation to be much more effective and longer lasting, because the skin had been physically lifted upwards and not just been stretched.

It was subsequently discovered that if more of the skin of the face was undermined (lifted or dissected) from the immediately underlying tissues and moved upwards and backwards and then fixed in position, the operation was even more successful. Because the skin was fixed into its new position it could not descend again to where it had been originally. The effect of a facelift could then be said to be permanent, in that after a facelift, a patient will always have the benefit of having had it done.

A woman who has a facelift at the age of 50 will still continue to age naturally. If she lives to be 90, however, she will not look as old as she would have done if she hadn't had the facelift. Many patients will undergo a repeat procedure long before they look as bad as their original preoperative appearance.

Between 1920 and 1950 more and more extensive dissections were undertaken. The incision grew from the original small crescent above the ear, to be extended in front of the ear, around the earlobe into the groove between the ear and the top of the neck, and back into the hair of the scalp of the back of the head for variable distances. The incisions behind the ear were useful for lifting the neck skin and jawline.

Because of the success of this procedure, in recent years the word 'facelift' has entered into the English language meaning 'any superficial improvement in appearance'.

The face is a complex structure consisting of several layers of different tissues. Deepest of all are the facial bones covered by several muscle layers. The muscles are covered by a layer of fat, which, in turn, is covered by an outside layer of skin.

In amongst the muscles and fat are the nerves, blood vessels and glands. Eventually surgeons realised that it wasn't just the skin that was aging and losing its elasticity, but all layers of the face. One of the problems with the early facelift approach was that if a surgeon pulled the skin up tightly to remove every wrinkle, the face took on a characteristic appearance that has been called the 'aging starlet' or 'wind-tunnel' look.

In the 1950s surgeons began to realise that if the muscles had stretched and drooped they could be lifted up as well as the skin, and thus achieve more natural-looking results. Because the muscles of the face are called the SMAS (Superficial Musculoaponeurotic System), lifting the muscles is called a SMAS-lift. Sometimes it is not necessary to lift the skin at all but just lift the muscle layer.

With the advent of liposuction in the 1970s, surgeons appreciated that repositioning the fat pads in the face would also contribute to a more successful and natural rejuvenation. Liposuction is used extensively in other areas of the body to sculpture unwanted pads of fat. In the face, the jowls and the double chin are unwanted pads of fat and they respond readily to liposuction. Some surgeons take the fat from the jowl area and under the chin and implant some of it into the nasolabial creases (nose to mouth lines) and into the lips. This is because it is a general feature of aging that, as well as losing elasticity and drooping, all of the tissues in the face reduce in volume. It is now possible partially to correct this in specific areas, such as the lips. The centre of the cheeks can also lose volume in some people, creating a gaunt look. Adding volume, either by the simple addition of fat, or, more successfully, by bulking out the cheek muscles by folding them over – a process known as plicating the SMAS – treats this.

In the last few years, some surgeons have resorted to the obsolete operation now renamed 'the minilift', where only the skin is lifted with a short incision, under local anaesthetic. Generally the results are short lived and disappointing, which is why this operation was abandoned in the first place.

A few surgeons are now doing what is called a thread lift, in which threads with tiny barbs are introduced under the skin (usually under local anaesthetic). When the threads are pulled backwards and upwards and tied to a strong part of the scalp the face is lifted a little. This technique is valid in cases where the face lifts readily. However, there is very little improvement if the face is significantly wrinkled or creased. It is also suspected that even the modest improvement will be rather short-lived.

How the Face Ages

The young individual has a firm, smooth face with only a few lines and wrinkles. The skin feels tight because it fits snugly over the fatty tissue, muscles and bones of the face.

As you age, the skin loses its elasticity, the muscles of the face lose tone and stretch and the fatty tissue shrinks in volume. The eventual result of this is that lines and wrinkles begin to appear and they become more prominent due to the effects of gravity and muscular action.

The most notable changes occur under the chin and upper neck (turkey neck and double chin), outer eyebrows (crow's feet), inner cheek area (jowl lines and furrows) and skin folds at the corner of the mouth.

A modern facelift operation attempts to lift and relocate all the structures of the face and neck that have sagged as a result of the aging process. This relocation of tissues conforms to the pattern seen in the younger individual thereby creating a more youthful appearance.

Two different types of aging are seen in the cheeks. In Type 1, the cheeks lose substance and become hollow; this is made much worse if the teeth are lost as well. In Type 2, the bulk of the cheek falls forwards and downwards producing a thick fold of tissue running from the side of the nose to the area below the jaw line where it ends as a jowl. In front of the jowl is a deep crease or fold referred to as the nasolabial crease or fold.

These two types of aging in the cheeks are now treated differently, so that the smooth curve that is a feature of a youthful cheek is restored, without having to pull the skin excessively tight. This avoids the unnatural, stretched, mask-like look that can occur with the traditional facelift. These new methods also make the facelift much more long lasting.

As you age, very fine lines appear where the skin is very close to the underlying muscle e.g. upper and lower eyelids, upper lip and forehead. The nose becomes sharper and longer in relation to the other facial features. This is because the nasal cartilages continue to grow while the overlying skin becomes thinner.

The rate of aging in a particular individual depends on a host of variables. Apart from inherited factors, other aspects that are important to the aging process are skin type, exposure to sunlight and wind, diet, alcohol consumption, smoking and stress. Chemicals applied to the skin such as aggressive make-up removers can also age sensitive skin. Chronic illness and its accompanying treatment can also play a major part.

The Aims of a Facelift

The purpose of a facelift operation is to raise and tighten the facial skin thereby eliminating or decreasing overhanging folds or lines. It also aims to correct the effects of aging on the deeper structures by tightening and relocating muscles that have stretched and drooped, and by removing redundant deposits of fat.

The standard facelift operation is effective in the neck, chin, cheeks and temporal regions i.e. the lower two thirds of the face and neck. The forehead and eyelid regions are not included in the standard operation and require separate procedures that may be combined with it.

It is not possible to eliminate every line, wrinkle or furrow in a facelift procedure. Prominent lines or wrinkles that remain will require additional treatment e.g. skin abrasion, filler injections with synthetic filling agents, or fat implants.

In some individuals a repeat procedure may be required within a year of the initial operation to gain maximum benefit, as some skin types, particularly in elderly patients, will not necessarily remain stretched after only one procedure.

Indications

To be suitable for this procedure you will have experienced some sagging of the facial tissues. Lifting the facial skin upwards and backwards with cupped hands will give an indication of the final result of the operation. If this manoeuvre gives a result that meets with your approval then the operation is likely to be successful. The facelift is one of the few operations where you can see the result, or get a good idea of what it will look like before you have it done.

There is no minimum age that qualifies a person to have the operation because the rate of aging is unique in every individual. Results are more striking when the signs of aging are very pronounced, hence less can be achieved in the younger patient with fewer signs of aging. It must be emphasised that risks and complications increase significantly with age.

A facelift has little or no effect on any surface changes of the skin due to aging. These are usually treated by ancillary procedures carried out at the same time as the main operation or separately e.g. laser resurfacing, dermabrasion or chemical peeling.

Preoperative considerations

Many patients undergoing this operation are elderly and may be suffering from a medical condition e.g. diabetes or hypertension. Any problems regarding fitness for surgery should be thoroughly assessed and treated beforehand.

If you are taking aspirin or other blood thinning medications you should desist from this if at all possible on account of the increased risk of postoperative bleeding (see page 49). Liaison with your attending physician or general practitioner will be of paramount importance.

Perhaps the most important single factor prior to facelift surgery concerns smoking. If you are a smoker you should cease smoking at least six weeks prior to surgery and for at least a month afterwards. The reason for this is that smoking reduces the blood supply to the skin flap, which can lead to flap necrosis (death of skin, ultimately resulting in an ugly scar), or impair and delay healing, leading to infection, particularly behind the ear. Smoking increases the rate of aging of the skin and is not compatible with looking younger for longer.

You should also not drink any alcohol for at least two weeks before the operation, because it can enhance postoperative bleeding (see page 49).

At the preliminary consultation the surgeon will carefully assess which of the many treatment possibilities will suit you best. This can be quite subjective. You could see several surgeons and gain the accurate impression that different alternative treatments are being suggested for your particular case.

Sometimes surgeons use different words to describe the same techniques. So you will need to pin down exactly what the surgeon proposes to do in your case, and compare it with your own ideas of what you think needs to be done. The old, basic facelift operation was a one-size-fits-all solution, but these days, with so many different treatments available, much more care has to be taken to match the treatment with your particular aims.

The operation

You will be admitted on the morning of surgery. A general or twilight anaesthetic (see 'Anaesthesia', pages 60–63) is usually administered. Because of this you should not have anything to eat or drink for some hours before the operation. The type of anaesthetic used will depend on the preference of the surgeon or patient. In nearly all cases the surgeon will inject local anaesthetic and adrenaline solution beneath the skin. This reduces bleeding, and therefore bruising afterwards, and postoperative pain. A facelift is not usually a painful experience for the patient. The local anaesthetic solution also makes the operation much easier to perform.

The incision begins in the temple behind the hairline, curving downwards to the top of the ear. The incision continues in the crease in front of the ear or slightly inside the ear canal behind the little protrusion of cartilage called the tragus. The incision used is specifically designed to be as inconspicuous as possible in any particular patient. The incision proceeds underneath the earlobe and then upwards in the groove behind the ear. It finally extends horizontally inside the hairline towards the back of the head.

The skin is then gently lifted (undermined or dissected) from the immediately underlying deeper tissues in order for it to be moved upwards. Skin undermining can be very extensive in the modern facelift, extending into the eyelids, over the cheeks to the corners of the mouth and then over the jaw line into the neck to meet the dissection from the opposite side in the midline under the chin.

In Type 1 cases (see page 76), the lost tissue of the cheek is reconstructed by folding the deeper tissues underneath the skin with appropriate stitches to recreate the smooth, natural fullness.

In Type 2 cases the redundant fat from the cheek folds and the jowls is removed by liposuction. The deep nose-to-mouth (nasolabial) folds or creases can be treated by implanting some of the fat that was removed from the cheek folds into them.

Excess fat in the neck that causes a double chin can also be removed by liposuction and the neck muscles tightened to produce a rejuvenation of the jaw line.

Some patients just have a droop of the muscle layers of the mid-face. In these cases it is possible to perform the procedure with a much shorter skin incision, and just pull up the muscle, a technique known as the 'S' lift. Because there is very little pull on the skin with this technique it is highly suitable for smokers, thereby reducing the chance of postoperative flap necrosis (see below) but unfortunately it is not appropriate for the majority of cases.

In a few cases where the muscles haven't sagged much and there is little or no jowl formation, but where the main problem is skin wrinkling, then radical undermining and lifting of the skin is all that is required. This technique is called a skin lift. It is basically the operation that was done between the wars, but again it is unsuitable for the majority of patients today.

Once the skin has been adequately undermined and all ancillary procedures to the deeper tissues completed, the skin is gently lifted upwards and backwards and stitched or stapled into the correct position after the excess skin has been trimmed. Most surgeons will insert drains for up to 48 hours. These drains – thin plastic tubes attached to a container maintaining a degree of suction – reduce the tendency for fluid to collect beneath the skin flap and help to reduce bruising, thereby speeding recovery (see page 41).

A modern facelift does not depend on all the structures of the face being lifted by being dragged upwards with the skin. Instead the deep structures are secured into their best position and the overlying skin then re-draped over them. This gives a much more natural and also longer-lasting effect.

During the healing process after the operation, the intention is that the skin will re-adhere to the deep facial structures in its new position. To enable this to happen, padded bandages are wrapped around at the end of the operation to apply a gentle pressure to the skin surface.

Postoperative management

All surgeons will manage their patients in their own particular way, based on their previous experience. However, the measures are likely to be as follows.

Strict bed rest is advised in the immediate postoperative period to reduce the risk of bleeding. Quick movements, bending, straining and lifting should be avoided initially, and, if possible, sneezing. Facial movement should be kept to a minimum. It is best to drink with a straw and avoid foods that require a lot of chewing.

Most patients do not find this procedure unpleasant. The commonest complaint is that of tightness of the face. Most surgeons usually prescribe sedatives initially as this reduces the risk of postoperative bleeding and bruising.

Patients are generally advised to sleep with the head elevated for a few days to reduce swelling. Swelling can be quite marked.

Bandages and drains are generally removed after 24 to 48 hours, and the hair is washed. Aspirin and alcohol are forbidden for at least two weeks before and after surgery (see page 49). Most patients are discharged from hospital after one or two days. A follow-up appointment is necessary after a week to ten days for review and suture removal.

Once you are back home after the operation, the hair should be washed frequently (every day) to help prevent wound infection, which is especially liable to occur behind the ear. It also keeps the stitches or the staples clean and makes them easier to remove.

Full recovery can take several months. Most patients should be fit to continue their normal activities in a few days and be confident to appear in public after about two weeks.

Postoperative events and complications

In addition to the postoperative complications mentioned (see 'Postoperative Concerns', pages 52–55) the following deserve specific attention.

Bleeding Bleeding can occur, as after any operation, and, if severe, the face swells up alarmingly, resulting in a collection of clotted blood under the skin flap called a haematoma. Less severe bleeds can be treated simply by drawing the blood out with a needle, or by massaging the collection of blood towards the incision line so that it can be evacuated.

A large expanding haematoma must be treated as an emergency as it can cause irreversible damage to the skin flap called 'flap necrosis' (see below). This is because the blood supply is cut off as a result of the severe tension in the skin flap produced by the expanding haematoma.

The patient has to be taken back to the operating theatre, where the wound is re-opened, the blood collection removed and the bleeding points sealed off. After successful treatment of a haematoma the recovery and the result of the operation should be as normal, although swelling may take longer to subside. The risk of haematoma formation is greater than normal if the patient has taken aspirin (or even a number of common dietary herbs – see Appendix, page 231) before the operation, or if they are overactive immediately after the operation.

Very small amounts of blood, which may not always be apparent after the operation, can produce prolonged lumps and irregularities during the recovery period. These usually settle, but it can take several weeks. Only rarely is further intervention necessary. Massaging the lumps twice a day for a few minutes helps them settle.

Bruising and swelling In most facelift cases there should be minimal bruising and swelling. If bleeding occurs under the skin flap after the drains have been removed there is a strong likelihood that bruising will take a few weeks to subside completely. Gentle massage with skin creams helps swelling and bruising to resolve.

Infection If wound infection occurs postoperatively, it most frequently occurs in the part of the wound that lies behind the ear. This is because this area of the skin flap has the lowest blood supply and because the groove behind the ear is most likely to get 'dirty' afterwards, thereby increasing the likely incidence of infection. Local hygiene (i.e. frequent washing) reduces the chance of infection.

Numbness This is common in the neck and cheek areas as well as around the ear. The numbness usually resolves within a few weeks. Very rarely, areas of numbness, especially on the ear, can be permanent. Some patients get a number of weird sensations in the cheeks during the recovery, but these usually all settle in time.

Change in previous hair pattern In all patients the hairline will be altered. This invariably occurs because the facial skin has been moved to a new position as a result of lifting it. The hairline in front of and behind the ear is largely affected. Facelifting is really the only common cause of a receding hairline in women.

Hair loss This can occur in the scalp adjacent to the incision lines. The hair growth usually recovers, but it can take many months. Sometimes the hair loss may be permanent and need further surgery to correct it (see 'The Treatment of Hair Loss', pages 200–213). Rarely, patchy areas of alopecia (hair loss) can occur in the temple, but this generally grows back in a few months.

Nerve injury On rare occasions, damage to any of the nerve branches that activate the facial muscles can produce weakness or paralysis of that muscle or group of muscles. This can result in asymmetrical facial movements, weakness or paralysis of the face.

Most cases of facial weakness following facelift surgery will resolve spontaneously. Rarely, further surgery to repair a nerve may be required in severe cases. Thankfully this complication is very rare in experienced hands.

Flap necrosis This is perhaps the worst complication of this procedure. It occurs where an area of the skin flap dies, ultimately resulting in an ugly scar. It is an extremely rare complication in experienced hands.

It occurs as a result of impairment to the blood circulation in the skin once it is lifted from the deeper tissues. The cause is often unknown but it is more common in heavy smokers or in association with a haematoma (see above). It is also seen in diabetics and many surgeons won't carry out facelifts on diabetic patients for this reason. Or, if they do, they will use techniques that don't put tension on the skin, such as the 'S' lift (see above, page 80).

In severe cases, further surgery may be required to improve the scarring but it will not completely eliminate it.

Scars Facelift incisions are placed where they are generally inconspicuous so scarring is not a major problem in facelift surgery. However, scars may get infected or stretch or thicken, requiring surgical revision (see 'Improving Unsightly Scars', pages 196–199) at a later stage.

Pigmentation This can occur over sites of bruising, and may be permanent.

Unnatural appearance or 'The Ventriloquist Dummy Look' The popularity of cosmetic surgery in recent years has yielded its own unique set of unfavourable circumstances. One of these is the increasing number of celebrities who have had one – or five! – too many facelifts, which ultimately give their faces a permanent pulled appearance, referred to by the authors as 'The Ventriloquist Dummy Look'.

Many patients are understandably concerned beforehand that they may end up looking like this. But this condition only occurs after the facial skin has suffered repeated, frequent facelifts, which eventually exhaust the skin's elasticity. It is highly unlikely to occur after one facelift or after a few well-spaced, expertly performed operations. It was much more commonly seen in the past, due to oft-repeated, too-tight skin lifts.

Asymmetry All human faces are not truly symmetrical. In the young, the bulky facial tissues generally disguise the bony asymmetry and this is also true when the tissues have sagged. However, when they have been pulled up and tightened, any underlying asymmetry may become more apparent. This should, however, still be well within normal range, and not obvious to an observer. It is surely compensated for by the general improvement in appearance.

Results

Patients who are good candidates for a facelift are likely to gain a very gratifying result. They can look years younger and this can be a great boost to their confidence. The improvement in appearance can be dramatic, and is usually even more so when combined with blepharoplasty (removal of eye bags) (see 'Eyelid Surgery', pages 94–99) and dermabrasion or other surface skin treatments to the upper lip (see page 91).

It is not possible to predict how long the beneficial effects of a facelift will last. In the initial stages, residual tissue swelling will enhance the result obtained from surgery. As tissue swelling gradually subsides, some original fine lines will reappear and the facial skin will gradually loosen.

It is important to appreciate that the aging process will continue after a facelift operation. Aging is a complex phenomenon and depends on many factors already discussed (see page 76–77). Because of the complexity and specificity of the aging process, the rate of aging is unique to every individual. In simple terms, however, a person who has had a facelift will not look as old after 10 years than if she hadn't had it done.

Having a facelift does not affect the rate of the aging process. The improvement gained – that is the lessening of the signs of aging compared to before the operation – is permanent in that the patient will not catch up with how they would have looked like had they not had it done. Sooner or later, however, depending on the factors mentioned above, the signs of aging will return. This can sometimes occur within a matter of months, but usually within a number of years. The operation can then be repeated.

TEMPORAL LIFT

This is really the upper half of a facelift. The incision is not carried around the ear but goes up high on the temporal scalp. It effectively removes crow's feet creases from the sides of the eyes and lifts the upper parts of the cheeks and outer parts of the eyebrows. It is often performed on relatively young patients who do not have any problems with the neck skin. It is often combined with eye-bag removal (see 'Eyelid Surgery', pages 94–99).

Brow Lift

The brow lift operation aims to flatten the vertical frown lines between the eyebrows and reduce the horizontal creases of the forehead. In addition it will lift the eyebrows to a more youthful position if they have sagged. This will give an open-eyed look, a feature of the young. It is often combined with upper blepharoplasty (see 'Eyelid Surgery', pages 94–99) and the combination often gives a better result than either operation alone. A brow lift can make all the difference to a sad, drawn look that is caused by deep forehead lines and low eyebrows. The results can last for many years. In general two types of procedure are performed routinely: the traditional or the endoscopic brow lift.

Traditional Brow Lift

The operation

A general or twilight anaesthetic (see 'Anaesthesia', pages 60–63) is usually administered, then local anaesthetic and adrenaline solution, as in a facelift (see page 79). The incision extends across the top of the head from ear to ear inside the hairline. The scalp is undermined (lifted away) from the incision line to the eyebrows and bridge of the nose. The muscles that produce the frown lines are weakened with appropriately placed incisions (cuts) and often some muscle is removed. The scalp is then stretched backwards and the excess scalp is trimmed. The incision is then sutured and is hidden because it lies well behind the hairline.

There is another, unusual technique for doing a browlift, that is useful in some cases. Here the incision is made just in front of the hairline all the way along. The forehead is undermined and the muscles weakened as usual to remove the frown lines. The skin of the forehead is redraped upwards and the overlap removed. The wound is then very carefully sutured. The advantage of this method is that there is no backwards movement of the hairline. The disadvantage is that there will be, in most cases, a visible scar just in front of the hair. This technique can be extended further, in that if the scalp is undermined, the hairline can be brought forwards. This will reduce a high forehead. The scar can be disguised by permanent make-up tattoo, or by transplanting a few hairs from the back of the head into the scar. In general this method is only successful in those patients who comb their hair forwards.

Postoperative events

Numbness and tingling This invariably occurs at the top of the head and can last for several weeks.

Hair loss This can occur around the incision and may be permanent.

Scar The scar may stretch and require a revision procedure at a later stage. Because the scar is entirely hidden in the hair, in most cases it can only be found if looked for.

Asymmetry This can occur resulting in one side being higher than the other. A revision procedure may be necessary.

Movement Immediately after the operation the forehead will have limited movement, but normal movement usually returns in a few weeks.

Endoscopic Brow Lift

Recent technological advances have introduced the wonders of 'keyhole surgery'. This revolutionary type of surgery uses an endoscope to perform its various functions.

An endoscope is made up of a tiny camera with a bright light fitted on the end of a long tube (the endoscope), which in turn is connected by a fibre optic cable to a television screen. A magnified image of what the camera is focusing on is displayed on the screen. Using specially designed instruments, which are inserted through tiny incisions, the surgeon can perform a wide range of surgical procedures that are monitored on the television screen, much like a video game.

Endoscopic surgery is gaining widespread popularity in many surgical specialities, including cosmetic surgery where it is mainly used for forehead and facial rejuvenation in selected cases. In practical terms, the endoscope has been found to be useful in the tightening up of parts of the face in relatively young patients, particularly the brow and forehead.

This technique requires proper patient selection and a great deal of skill and expertise by the surgeon in order to achieve consistently good results.

The operation

The procedure is usually performed under sedation or general anaesthetic, and local anaesthetic is injected under the skin to be lifted. Usually five small incisions are used.

Specially designed instruments are passed through these incisions and lift the scalp from the skull, cutting and weakening the appropriate muscles to reduce the frown lines and finally fix the elevated scalp to its new site. The endoscope is also passed through one of these incisions and allows the surgeon to see what he is doing.

The elevation is maintained by suspending the scalp on sutures that pass through the tissues near the eyebrows and are then attached further back to the bone of the skull, either by drilling small holes in the bone or by screwing in special fixation devices.

No skin is removed with this technique.

Postoperative events

The same sequelae that occur after traditional browlift (see pages 85–86) can occur after endoscopic browlift, except that the small scars are unlikely to stretch.

Result

Because endoscopic surgery involves much less invasive surgery than the traditional brow lift (see above), there is less disturbance to facial tissues and a more rapid recovery from surgery. The longer and more noticeable scars of a traditional brow lift are also avoided. However, the technique is more suited to younger patients where there is less need to excise much skin. Also, the permanence of the lift may be more limited. Its best use is in those (generally male) patients who have a receding hairline, where the scar of the traditional or open brow lift would show, and where the limited result and less permanent result are a worthwhile trade-off for invisible scarring.

DOUBLE-CHIN REMOVAL

In some people fat is deposited beneath the jawline at an early age to give a double chin. In most cases, however, an excess deposit of fat under the chin is associated with aging, or simply being overweight. In addition loose skin under the chin and neck together with vertical bands that run from the chin to the base of the neck create the 'turkey neck' deformity.

In young people with a double chin the excess of fat can be removed by liposuction alone. Where there is loose skin, liposuction has to be supplemented with skin and muscle tightening, usually achieved with a facelift (see pages 74–84).

THE CHEEKS

One of the most obvious signs of aging is the increasing hollowness of the cheeks. Facial fullness is diminished by the reduction of fat, muscle weakness and loss of teeth, associated with the aging process of the face (see pages 76–77). The excess skin of the cheeks is drawn inwards and thrown into folds.

The problem with losing the teeth is that the gums shrink when they are not supporting the teeth. When dentures are fitted on these thin gums they cannot be made up to be the same height as the teeth were originally. In extreme old age the loss of tissue between the nose and the chin produces the characteristic witch-like appearance.

Several procedures are available to enhance the projection of the cheeks. Young people who want bigger cheekbones obviously want an operation that is going to be permanent. The insertion of cheek implants may be more suitable for them than the use of synthetic fillers. Some of the fillers introduced recently are designed to last several years, however, and, as they give a more subtle result than an implant, and are also generally a good deal cheaper, they can be a good alternative.

Cheek Implants

The height and projection of the cheekbones can be altered by the insertion of specially designed, silicone cheek implants. Cheek implants are silicone plastic shapes designed to rest on the patient's own cheekbones. These are usually inserted via a small incision in the mouth, but can also be inserted as part of a facelift, or using a small incision just beneath the eyelashes of the lower eyelid.

The operation

Cheek implant insertion, known as malarplasty, is usually performed as a day case under general anaesthetic. Local anaesthetic is injected, as in other facial surgery, for the same reasons (see page 79). The usual approach is via a small incision in the mouth near the gum of the canine tooth on each side. A pocket is opened up over the cheekbone that just fits the size and shape of the implant. It is important that the implant is a snug fit in its pocket so that it cannot move about.

After the implants are inserted they are carefully checked for correct position and symmetry and the wound closed. For a day or two, extreme facial movements should be avoided. Great care must be taken in order to allow for optimum healing of the incisions inside the mouth. The swelling and bruising are usually minimal and only last for a few days.

Postoperative events

Malposition   Cheek implants can move out of position, resulting in an asymmetrical appearance to the face. This is more likely to happen during the early postoperative phase, or after a direct blow to the cheeks, or sometimes as a result of sustained deforming pressure, such as leaning the face on a hand while studying or reading.

Asymmetry   The cheekbones are never truly symmetrical and sometimes adding an implant exaggerates this. This would have to be carefully evaluated by the surgeon preoperatively. Grossly asymmetrical cheekbones may make the surgeon proceed only with great caution, or render the patient unsuitable for treatment.

Infection   This can occur in the postoperative period. The implant has to be removed and the infection effectively treated before re-insertion of the implant.

Odd sensations or numbness in the face   This can occur immediately after the operation and, sometimes, for a few weeks after. This is caused by minor nerve damage during the insertion of the implant. During the healing phase facial sensation should return to normal.

Visible implant   With aging and its associated thinning of all the facial tissues, after many years there may be less tissue covering the implant than when the surgery was first performed. In such cases the outline of the implant may become visible. This could be corrected by trimming the implant or by thickening the covering tissues during a facelift. Simply removing an implant that has been in position for a long time is likely to leave a visible dent. Sometimes synthetic fillers applied around the margin of the implant can be used to soften the edge.

Results

Cheek implants can produce a dramatic improvement in suitable cases and the result will be permanent. Higher cheekbones tend to make people more photogenic. The insertion of cheek implants is one of the rare operations in cosmetic surgery that is easily reversible. The implants can generally be removed quite easily through the same approach used for their insertion. If they were inserted through the mouth there would be no visible scar from either the insertion or the removal. However, if the implants have been in place for several years, removing them without doing any other treatment to compensate would probably leave a dent.

As Part of a Face Lift

The loss of the fullness of the cheeks can be improved by doubling over the cheek tissues under the skin, which can be done as part of a facelift in special cases. This produces a much more attractive rounded shape to the cheek which is virtually permanent. However, this does not produce as dramatic a difference in accentuating the height of the cheekbones as inserting synthetic cheek implants (see above).

Autologous (own-body) fat implants

Injecting autologous (the patient's own) fat into the hollow of the cheek or over the cheekbones can be performed to replace volume lost due to aging. This technique is also effective in correcting minor discrepancies in the shape and size of the two cheeks.

The results are semi permanent. Initially some of the fat will be dissolved and absorbed relatively quickly (within a few weeks) but the fat that 'takes' and continues to thrive will only gradually be absorbed. This might eventually necessitate a repeat maintenance procedure to replenish the absorbed tissue. The fat lasts much better in the hollow of the cheek than over the bone but, unfortunately, the volume of fat that can be implanted at any one time is quite limited. This is because, in order to survive, the transplanted fat has to establish an adequate blood supply to ensure its long term survival. Failure to achieve this will result in the fat being dissolved and absorbed.

If the fat implant is put too near the skin and in too great a quantity, an uneven puckering can result. This is another reason for the surgeon not to be too ambitious with this technique. Surgeons experienced in fat transfer usually get consistently good results with very few adverse effects.

Synthetic injectable fillers

There is an increasing number of semi-permanent injectable fillers available, which can be used to augment the cheeks when they have become hollow or over the cheekbones themselves to act as a malarplasty (see above, pages 88–89). They have to be used with some caution when augmenting hollow cheeks, because a large mass of filler won't move in the same way as natural body tissues when smiling or laughing. However, they can make a significant difference, and are useful in correcting small asymmetries.

THE LIPS

The aging process affects the lips, just like the rest of the body. The upper lip becomes less bulky with vertical creases, known as 'barcode lines'. These problems are made much worse by smoking, and also by the loss of teeth. The vertical lines are very effectively treated by dermabrasion (see page 110–113), a deep chemical peel or by laser resurfacing, which can be combined with a facelift. The loss of bulk is effectively treated by synthetic fillers or by autologous fat implants (see above).

Lip Enlargement (Cheiloplasty)

One of the features of aging is that the opening of the mouth moves downwards. When a young girl smiles she generally shows the fronts of her top teeth. In middle age she is likely to show the gap between the upper and lower teeth. When the elderly smile, they often show the fronts of the lower teeth. This process is due to the lengthening and thinning of the upper lip. Often the height of the pink or vermilion part of the lip reduces as well.

In the cheiloplasty operation, a strip of skin is removed from the lip margins. When the wound is closed it rolls the lip outwards so that the lip pouts more. It also increases the height of the vermilion in the upper lip and shortens the distance between the base of the nose and the vermilion margin. It produces a scar along the upper border of the vermilion, where there is a natural line anyway. The scar can be easily disguised with lipstick or lip liner, or it can be treated with permanent make-up if it is unsightly. Both upper and lower lips can be enlarged in this way, but the operation is more successful in the upper lip.

This operation can be very successful in young people who have a long upper lip that covers their teeth when they smile, or those who have a thin, mean-looking upper lip with a low vermilion margin – so it is not performed because of aging alone. It would be unsuitable for a patient who already has a gummy smile, showing the gums and upper parts of the upper teeth.

Cheiloplasty can be easily done under local anaesthetic as a day case. A dressing is necessary for a week, but after the dressing has been removed lipstick can be applied straight away. This is an area extremely resistant to infection and the wound will be impervious to bacteria after a week.

Lip Filling

If the patient desires her lips to be fuller, then either an injectable filling agent or a permanent implant can be used. If the upper lip is already too long and covers the teeth, a cheiloplasty (see above) is a better procedure, as lip filler will probably lengthen the lip. There are three sites in which it is possible to inject the filler, and they each have different indications:

1. Along the vermilion margin. This exaggerates the demarcation between the vermilion and the normal skin and makes the upper lip pout more. This effect is popularly known as the Paris Lip.
2. Into the vermilion itself, to create bigger, fleshier lips.
3. Deep into the main body of the upper lip to augment the lip when the normal youthful bulk has been lost by aging.

Most fillers don't last very long when they are used in the lips because the area is so mobile. Fillers designed to be long lasting in other areas of the body have a tendency to form hard lumps when placed just beneath the lip skin, especially the vermilion. Often the lips don't move properly and look odd when smiling and talking if too much filler is injected. Putting filler in the lower lip is much more problematic than inserting it into the upper lip because the augmented lip may not be supported well. It can thus fall downwards and forwards, spoiling the effect.

Both natural and synthetic implants can be used to enhance lip size. Natural implants can be obtained by using skin or scar tissue from the patient or from prepared cadaver skin. This type of implant is called a dermal graft. Cadaver implants are specially prepared to minimise the chances of rejection by the recipient. They are available prepacked and sterilised for immediate use, thereby precluding the need to harvest tissue from the patient.

A previous scar from a patient (e.g. an appendix scar) can be excised (removed) from a patient and the resulting defect sutured. The excised scar is then de-epithelialised (superficial skin layer removed) leaving a strip of tissue consisting of skin dermis and scar tissue. This tissue can then be suitably trimmed and shaped to be inserted along the upper and lower lip margins to enhance their size. The procedure is usually performed under local anaesthetic as a day case. Cadaver implants are inserted using a similar technique.

Stab incisions are made at the extremities of the upper or lower lips. The implant is threaded into the lip at the desired depth using a specially designed surgical instrument.

Postoperative discomfort, bruising and swelling are short lived and not usually severe. Antibiotics are routinely prescribed to reduce the chance of infection.

Although this procedure is usually very successful and results long lasting, the implant can occasionally be broken down by the body and absorbed very quickly after only a few weeks. The reason is unclear but is more likely to happen if infection occurs soon after the procedure.

Synthetic implants, in the form of threads or suture material or special plastic implants have also been used a lot in the past in the lips, but they are less popular these days, simply because there is a greater and more effective choice of injectable fillers. Most of the synthetic implants suffer from the disadvantage that, if they are of any significant size, they can be felt by the patient and sometimes even seen by other observers. They can also eventually displace.

Lip Reduction

Oversized, thick lips that pout too much can be reduced by taking out an appropriate strip of mucosa (the lining surface of the lip on the inside of the mouth) and underlying lip tissue from inside the mouth. This rotates the lips inwards, towards the teeth. This operation is most commonly performed on people of black African descent. Because the scars are inside the mouth they are hidden from view. It can be done under local anaesthetic as a day case.

The swelling immediately after this operation can be quite dramatic and can last for months. When the swelling has gone down the lips will be significantly smaller. There is a limit to how much can be removed however, because if too much is taken away the lips will not close properly. The operation works well on both upper and lower lips.

After this operation it is likely that the lips will be numb for a while. Take care with hot food and drinks. Sensation should return to normal within a few weeks.

Eyelid Surgery (Blepharoplasty)

EYELID SURGERY

Aging around the eyes is associated with the formation of excess skin folds and eyebags. The slow loss of skin elasticity significantly affects the upper eyelids. In the young the skin is stretchy enough to take up the slack when the eyes are open. With aging, the skin is unable to do this, so when the eyes are open a fold of skin forms above the upper eyelid crease. In the very elderly this fold can fall over the eyelid and interfere with vision. Simple trimming of this excess skin can improve vision.

With aging the brow moves downwards (see pages 85–87), so that the eyebrows come to lie below the bony brow ridge. This exaggerates the effect of the excess skin of the eyelid itself.

As part of aging, the eyeballs themselves recede slightly into the orbits (the eye sockets). The result of the eyeballs moving backwards is to push the fat around them forwards where it forms soft lumps under the skin called eyebags. The fat from behind the eyes also comes forward due to the stretching of the membrane that holds it in place. In some cases this fatty protrusion is inherited and becomes noticeable at a much younger age than usual.

Eye-bags are especially seen in the inner or medial parts of the upper eyelid and along the length of the lower eyelid. Eye-bag formation increases progressively with aging.

Excess skin folds and eye-bags cause eye shadow make-up to become smudged at the lid folds.

The aim of the surgery
The aim of surgery is to reduce the excess skin and flatten the eye-bags. There is no simple surgical technique that will restore the position of the eyeball to its youthful location. Before surgery it is recommended to have

an eye test to assess vision as well as tear production. The laxity of both lids is also noted, as this will affect the operative technique.

The operation
You will be admitted to the clinic on the morning of surgery. The procedure is usually performed under sedation and local anaesthesia, although a general anaesthetic is sometimes preferable for a nervous patient.

In the upper lid the incision is made in the lid crease. In the lower lid, the incision starts at the outer side in a crow's foot crease and extends under the eyelashes. No patient's eyes or the creases around them are completely symmetrical, and the surgeon has to decide whether to make symmetrical incisions or use the pre-existing creases. Through these incisions, excess fat, skin and, if necessary, muscle can be appropriately removed.

Sutures are usually removed three to five days after the operation.

In cases where the lower eyelids have good skin tone but an excess of protruding fat, the surgeon may choose to perform a 'transconjunctival blepharoplasty'. Here the lower eyelid is pulled forwards and an incision is made on the inner surface of the lid, which allows access to the fatty pockets of the lower eyelids. The excess fat can thus be removed, and no stitches are required. If the lower eyelid skin has already lost tone, then this approach will increase the wrinkles, so it is usually done in young patients only.

Some surgeons treat the skin with laser or dermabrasion at the same time as performing this transconjunctival removal of the eye-bag. But, if there is a significant amount of spare skin, most surgeons will opt for the formal skin-excision technique.

Postoperative events

Swelling and bruising Swelling and bruising around the eyes is inevitable. The bruising usually subsides within 10 days. Minor degrees of swelling may persist for a few weeks afterwards. Scars can usually be camouflaged by make-up after a few days. The scars will fade in time and become perceptible only on very close scrutiny.

Watery eyes This can occur for a few days postoperatively and generally subsides spontaneously.

Dark skin Preoperative pigmentation of the lower eyelid skin will not be improved following this procedure. Indeed the condition may become more pronounced.

Bleeding Occasionally a small collection of blood may accumulate under the skin and may need to be evacuated. This can be acheived either by aspiration using a needle or, if that fails, the wound will have to be opened again and the clot removed. Persistent bleeding in the deeper tissues of the orbit may temporarily increase the pressure in the orbit. This is extremely rare and may require inpatient treatment, although a further operation is usually unnecessary.

Drooping of the upper eyelid This is caused by unnoticed accidental trauma to the muscle that elevates the eyelid. A further operation may be necessary to correct this problem. This is in complete contrast to drooping associated with loose skin in the first instance. Fortunately this complication is extremely rare in experienced hands and repair is usually very successful.

Drooping of the lower eyelid (Ectropion) This sometimes occurs in the immediate postoperative period as a result of swelling, and usually rectifies itself in a few days. Sometimes the condition can arise as a result of excess skin resection (removal) at operation or from contraction of the tissues during healing. Occasionally a further surgical procedure is required to improve the situation.

Scleral (the white of the eye) show In nearly all cases the lower lid won't rise as high up the eyeball as it did before. In a few cases the white of the eye can be seen below the coloured part (i.e. the iris) resulting in a stare. Some people have this condition naturally without surgery. It sometimes occurs after surgery for no apparent reason, but it is generally attributed to removing too much tissue from the lower eyelid.

This situation usually occurs when the surgeon is trying to remove all the wrinkles in the eyelid. Most surgeons accept that eyelid surgery has to err on the side of caution. If a surgeon is being a bit over ambitious then scleral show becomes more likely. It can also be a late complication as a result of the scar contracting in the lower lid. Scleral show is often seen temporarily for a while after the operation and is due to the swelling, but it usually self-corrects. It is helped if the patient pushes the eyelid up carefully with a finger during the postoperative period. They should do this several times daily until the condition is resolved, which is usually within a few days, but can take much longer.

Hollowed-eye look If the surgeon removes all the protruding fat, or worse, takes too much away, a hollowed look results. This is due to thinning of the tissues in the area, which is a natural result of aging, so it may not be avoidable in all cases. Because of this it is usual for the surgeon to be cautious in removing the excess fat. It is better to leave a little excess fat than to remove too much.

Change of shape Sometimes eyelid surgery causes the eyes to be rounder in shape than they were before. This is most likely to happen if a considerable amount of skin is removed.

Inability to close the eyes completely This can sometimes occur in the immediate postoperative period and treatment with eye drops is all that is required before the condition rectifies itself. In the rare instance that too much tissue has been removed a further procedure may be required.

Postoperative wrinkling This can occur if the bags alone have been removed and the excess skin left forms creases or wrinkles. This is particularly more likely to happen with 'transconjunctival blepharo-plasty' (see above, page 95) where a tightening procedure was not performed. Further surgery may be required to improve the situation.

Infection This can occur in the outer coating of the eye (conjunctivitis), the incision lines (wound infection) and eyelid margins (blepharitis). These infections will require appropriate treatment, usually with ointments.

Loss of eyelashes This is very rare. The lashes however usually regenerate.

Dry eyes Patients already suffering from this rare condition called the Dry Eye Syndrome (keratoconjunctivitis sicca) should inform the surgeon, as eyelid surgery may worsen the situation. Many elderly patients don't produce as much tear fluid as when they were young, and they may notice that the eyes seem dryer after blepharoplasty.

Asymmetry Many patients who complain that their eyes are different from each other after the operation are noticing for the first time a situation that actually existed before. If the asymmetry has been caused by the operation it can usually be corrected without difficulty.

Conjunctival chemosis Sometimes fluid can collect under the conjunctiva (covering layer) in the lower part of the eye to look like a blister or bubble on the surface of the eye. The cause of this is largely unknown but is likely to be the result of impaired lymphatic drainage to the surface covering of the eye. Usually, this condition rectifies itself spontaneously after a few days and treatment with drops is all that is required. If it persists however, referral to an ophthalmic surgeon may be indicated. Treatment consists of aspirating the fluid with a very fine needle or rarely an operation to open the blister so that the fluid can be drained.

Blindness This extremely rare complication causes concern to many patients. Although this complication has been reported in the medical literature the reason for it is unclear. It has not occurred in our experience.

Postoperative management

Alcoholic drinks and aspirin-containing drugs should be avoided for two weeks pre- and post-operatively. Quick movements should be avoided initially. Individual surgeons will have their preferences with respect to treating bruising and swelling.

Cold water compresses can be applied to the eyes for five minutes every hour for the first 12 hours, thereafter three times daily for three days in order to reduce the swelling and bruising.

Ointment and eye drops can be applied at the discretion of the surgeon. Contact lenses should not be worn for at least two weeks afterwards. Normal activities can be resumed in seven to 14 days.

Result

The result of a successful blepharoplasty can be dramatic and extremely pleasing for the patient, as well as long lasting. The best result is obtained if a facelift is performed at the same time. Eyelids without creases and bags will look much younger and the eyes will often look larger.

Surgery of the Oriental Eye

The essential difference between a Caucasian and Oriental upper eyelid is that the former has a transverse fold or crease above the eyelashes. Many oriental women would like to have 'Western' eyes and this operation is extremely popular in Asia.

The operation

The operation is usually performed under sedation and local anaesthesia. Through a transverse (horizontal) incision in the upper lid, a fold is created by stitching part of the muscle that elevates the upper eyelid into the deeper layer of the skin. Several operations have been devised to produce this effect, and the techniques used vary with different surgeons.

Postoperative management

Postoperative management is along the same lines as for upper blepharoplasty.

The Treatment of Facial Lines, Wrinkles and Furrows

It must be emphasised that successful treatment of lines, wrinkles and furrows depends on their site, severity and extent, as well as the preference of surgeon and patient alike. At the first consultation all the possible options should be discussed and considered. Some patients ask for treatment for wrinkles, but should really be considering more formal surgery, such as a facelift (see pages 74–84) or blepharoplasty (see 'Eyelid Surgery', pages 94–99). Just treating the wrinkles and furrows in a patient who really needs a facelift can often lead to disappointment.

At the consultation stage, a cosmetic surgeon is likely to inform the patient of this fact, but, unfortunately, many treatments for wrinkles are carried out by non-medically qualified personnel, and it may take a lot of time and money before the patient realises that the treatment is ineffective.

Quite often injectable fillers can be used in conjunction with extensive surgery to produce the best result. The last few years have seen a massive increase in the number of treatments available for reducing facial lines, wrinkles and furrows. These treatments can be divided into the following categories:

1. Injectable fillers:
   - Semi-permanent (temporary) including fat transfer
   - Permanent
   - Implants which are permanent but removable
2. Implants: (inserted surgically under the skin. They are permanent but removable)

3. Skin Resurfacing:
  • Dermabrasion
  • Chemical Peels:
   a) Superficial
   b) Deep
  • Laser
4. Muscle Denervation (Botox®) treatment

INJECTABLE FILLERS

In the last few years, an increasing number of injectable, wrinkle-filling agents (fillers) have been developed and approved for use in Europe. Many of these fillers consist of chemicals that are found naturally in the supporting framework of the skin, such as various types of collagen or hyaluronic acid. Others are synthetic, such as microscopic plastic beads, or crystals of hydroxyapatite, a chemical that is found in bones. Some fillers contain both natural and synthetic components.

The majority of these fillers are classified as being semi-permanent or temporary i.e. they are gradually degraded and absorbed by the body.

Permanent injectable fillers have been used for many years particularly for the lower part of the face. It is currently maintained by most medical practitioners that permanent injectable fillers should *not* be used to treat facial lines and wrinkles because of possible long-term complications.

The first permanent filler was liquid silicone, which is very well tolerated by the body and lasts virtually forever. Unfortunately it has a tendency to drift slowly in the tissue. If it is injected in the base of a crease, five years later it is likely that it will have travelled up the sides of the crease, making the crease much deeper and more difficult to treat. Liquid paraffin has also been tried in addition to silicone but there were a lot of problems with chronic inflammation, which made the treated creases become permanent red lines. Both these permanent fillers have long since been abandoned, and modern fillers are much safer and more effective.

There is little doubt that facial fillers will further escalate in popularity in the near future. Safer, longer lasting ones are being developed. The current safe, tried and tested semi-permanent fillers usually last no more than three months and patients are prevented from seeking regular future 'top-ups' because of the pain of the injections and the related expense.

Temporary Fillers

Ideally, a temporary wrinkle filler should not cause allergies, not move from its original placement, be safe, be injectable through a very fine needle to minimise discomfort, be undetectable once in place, be long lasting, and of minimal cost. At present no temporary fillers satisfy all these criteria completely.

There are currently over 200 different temporary fillers available. Not all have been adequately tested or approved by their national regulatory bodies. The commonest and most approved ones currently used in the UK are described below. New fillers are constantly being developed and introduced.

On every occasion when the skin is pricked with a needle, there is a small chance of introducing infection or of puncturing a blood vessel, which will lead to unexpected bruising and swelling. Some fillers have a propensity to produce allergic reactions in sensitive people. If this describes you, then you need to have a skin test before the treatment is started.

There are available a large number of other fillers besides those we describe below. However, many of them have not been in use for very long, and thus we currently reserve judgement on their efficacy. The fillers we describe here have been in use for some time and have a proven track record.

Collagen

Collagen is a natural protein found throughout the body and is the main component of skin. Collagen fibres form 75 per cent of the total connective tissue fibres found in the dermis. Elastic fibres run parallel or obliquely to the collagen fibres and give skin its elasticity. A young person has a high content of elastic fibres; hence the skin is supple and springs back easily when stretched. It is analogous to the presence of lycra® fibres in a piece of clothing. Many anti-aging treatments attempt to stimulate the formation of new collagen and elastic fibres.

With aging, the collagen and elastic fibres are gradually diminished or destroyed resulting in the skin losing its elasticity and becoming loose. As a consequence, smiling, frowning and the effects of gravity result in the formation of lines and wrinkles. Excessive exposure to sunlight and smoking help to accelerate this process.

The damaged collagen can be replenished by injecting highly purified animal collagen, which the body accepts as its own and incorporates into the skin, filling in the wrinkles and smoothing the surface of the skin. It becomes a functioning part of the skin and even stimulates new natural collagen formation.

It is well known that small flakes of skin are constantly being shed from its surface to be replaced by new skin, which grows to the surface from the adjacent deeper tissue. Less well known is the fact that *all* tissues in the body undergo this gradual degradation and renewal process at different rates. As a result, if collagen is injected into the skin it will gradually be degraded and removed. This is why collagen injections have a limited lifespan and need to be repeated in order to maintain the desired effect.

There are several different types and strengths of collagen available. Each type is designed either for a specific area or for a particular kind of skin crease, wrinkle or fold. Some collagen preparations, although they are natural products, are chemically treated to resist the degrading process and last a bit longer after injection. A consultation with your surgeon will determine how best to treat you, in particular the type and amount of collagen required as well as to assess the likely result and your suitability for treatment.

Before treatment can begin, a small amount of collagen is injected into the skin of the forearm as an allergy test. Ninety-seven per cent of patients will show no reaction to the skin test and can proceed with treatment. The result of the test is assessed after four weeks. Assuming there is no reaction to the test dose, the treatment consists of a series of tiny injections into the wrinkles and is performed as an outpatient procedure.

Like the body's own collagen, the new collagen will gradually be depleted or absorbed by the body and further 'top-ups' will be required at intervals. As there are many skin types and several different factors involved it is not possible to predict accurately how long the effects of each injection will last in any particular individual. In most cases 'top-ups' are required every few months.

It is often said that the lifespan of a skin filler at a particular site is inversely proportional to the amount of movement it is subjected to. Thus the more movement it is subjected to the shorter it will last. This explains why fillers often do not last very long in the lips.

Hyaluronic acid gel

Hyaluronic acid is a natural material present in all connective tissue. It has been developed as a filling agent similar to collagen and is used in the same way, but a skin test is not required because allergy to it is extremely rare.

The commercially available products are either extracted from rooster combs or more recently as a synthetic (manufactured in the laboratory and therefore of non-animal origin) formulation that is claimed to offer longer-lasting results. This product is also available in different strengths, which are recommended to treat different problems.

Synthetic hyaluronic acid Restylane® gel, (Produced by Q-Med) is a stable and biodegradable synthetic hyaluronic acid.

After injecting it into skin, the gel binds with water and remains in place for many months, because the rate of absorption into the tissue of hyaluronic acid is much slower than collagen. Being synthetic and non-animal in origin there is no risk of transmitting disease or developing an allergic reaction in those sensitive to common foods such as beef, chicken and eggs.

In the last few years, Q-Med has extended its product range. The different products available at the present time are classified according to their particle size. The smaller the particle size the less viscous the material and the more suitable it is for treating the finest lines and wrinkles without producing long-lasting lumps. The larger the particles the more suitable the product is for treating the deeper lines and wrinkles. The current product range includes:

- Restylane Touch (approximately 500,000 particles per ml.) is used to treat fine superficial lines e.g. vertical upper lip (smokers') lines and crows feet. It should be injected into the upper dermis.

- Restylane (approximately 100,000 particles per ml.) is used to treat naso-labial lines, oral commissures as well as enhancing lip definition. It should be injected into the mid dermis.

- Restylane Perlane (approximately 10,000 particles per ml.) is used to treat deep wrinkles or folds e.g. naso-labial furrows, oral commissures, lip augmentation. It should be injected into the mid to deep dermis.

- Restylane Sub Q (approximately 1,000 particles per ml.) is used for chin, cheek and mid face augmentation. It should be injected deep to the skin.

Duration of action All Restylane preparations last for several months, but none are permanent. Restylane Sub Q should last over a year. How long each preparation lasts is very variable and depends on inherent genetic factors, age, skin type, lifestyle, and muscle activity, as well as on the injection technique employed.

With Restylane Sub Q injections, the area to be treated will have to be numbed first. With the other preparations, injections can be performed without using a numbing agent, or by using local anaesthetic creams or nerve blocks to numb the area beforehand. Afterwards, temporary swelling, redness and discomfort can occur. In extremely rare cases an allergic reaction can occur. It is possible, but unlikely, that infection can be caused by the injection, in which case the injection site may be red for weeks. Bleeding in the skin caused by the needle puncturing a blood vessel can produce significant temporary bruising and swelling.

Non-synthetic hyaluronic acid

- Hylaform (another form of stabilised hyaluronic acid) is derived from rooster combs and currently comes in three forms: Hylaform Fineline, Hylaform and Hylaform Plus. The mode and duration of action is similar to Restylane. As with Restylane, a preliminary skin test is not required.

Other synthetic fillers

- Radiesse® (formally called Radiance) is a synthetic dermal filler. The main ingredient is an inorganic substance called calcium hydroxylapatite (CaHa), which is the same in composition as the mineral portion of human bone and teeth. It contains no animal products and therefore no skin testing is necessary.

  When injected into the deep dermis it provides a scaffolding into which the body's own tissue can grow and add volume. It is used primarily in soft tissue augmentation e.g. lip and cheek enhancement, as well as filling deep skin folds and wrinkles.

  The product can be injected through a fine needle with or without topical anaesthetic or nerve block. Results can last for over a year. Complications include bruising and nodule (lump) formation especially in the lips.

- Reviderm Intra is another non-animal, synthetic, semi-permanent, injectable dermal implant for lip augmentation and the treatment of wrinkles.

  It consists of dextran microbeads suspended in hyaluronic acid (see above). In addition it is slowly biodegradable for long-lasting effects, stimulates the growth of connective tissue in the dermis, is non-allergenic and non-migratory (it doesn't move or spread from the injection site).

It is injected into the deep dermis with a fine needle and is commonly used to treat naso-labial folds, glabellar frown lines (the glabella is the part of the forehead above and between the eyebrows) and other facial wrinkles. After injection the area should be carefully massaged with the fingers by the surgeon to ensure the product is evenly distributed into the tissue, so as to avoid the possibility of forming lumps. A second or third injection may be necessary after four to eight weeks. Effects can last for one-and-a-half to two years.

Results from temporary fillers

Usually creases are reduced in depth rather than eradicated entirely.

All fillers can have adverse effects. Some need skin testing first, and even this does not guard against possible delayed complications. There are still many fillers being widely used that are still being evaluated. Because filler injections are simple to administer and are classed as being minimally or non invasive, an increasing number of medical practitioners from different specialities, and even dentists and nurses are regularly performing these treatments. Because semi-permanent fillers will eventually degrade or absorb, the chances of serious complications are greatly reduced.

Fat Transfer

The transfer of fat has been extensively employed for many years to fill out a variety of contour defects on the surface of the body. Fat transfer involves transplanting fat cells (containing the fat) and is regarded as a type of graft. In their new position they continue as before to absorb and store fat. Fat transfer is especially useful in correcting facial defects from whatever cause. The abundant blood supply of the face makes it an ideal area to support and maintain the viability – the ability to continue to live and thrive – of free transplanted fat cells. In addition, as they are the body's own tissue, there is no danger of rejection.

.The commonest cause of a facial defect is the aging process. Here there is usually a loss of fat under the skin at various sites, the commonest being the furrows that develop from the base of the nose to the outer edges of the lip, also known as naso-labial creases. Fat transfer works very well in this site and it is also useful for increasing the volume of the upper lip.

Technique
Fat transfer is usually performed as part of another operation, such as a facelift. When it is done on its own it can be done on an outpatient basis under local anaesthetic. The donor and recipient sites are numbed with local anaesthetic.

Using specially designed cannulae (small, narrow, blunt surgical tubes) attached to a syringe, the fat cells are painlessly aspirated (harvested) from the donor site into a syringe. This fat is then washed and carefully prepared for transfer into the recipient site. Donor fat is commonly obtained from fat in the stomach, thighs or buttocks.

The prepared harvested fat cells are then injected into the numbed recipient site using another specially designed blunt cannula. Sutures are not required because the incisions are so small.

Postoperative events
Bruising and swelling can occur for a few days. Infection is rare.

Results
About two thirds of the transplanted fat will be absorbed soon after transfer and within about six weeks of the procedure. Some will be absorbed at a later stage, while the remainder will 'take' and continue to thrive as normal living tissue. It is not possible, however, to predict accurately how much fat will 'take', and a second procedure is sometimes required within a few weeks.

Because only a small proportion of the volume of the transplanted fat is going to last more than a few weeks, it is customary to inject rather more than is actually required.

Unfortunately, if the surgeon tries to be over-ambitious with this technique the result tends to be disappointing because large volumes of fat cells do not establish an adequate blood supply and so perish. The correct technique is to inject only small amounts at a time. Many surgeons over the years have tried to use this technique to increase the size of the breasts, but because of this limitation it is quite unsuitable for this purpose. A small graft of fat cells that would make a very pleasing improvement in the lips would have a negligible effect in a breast.

The stable result, seen after six weeks or so, can last for several years.

Permanent Fillers
Permanent injectable fillers have been used for many years, particularly in the lower part of the face. Ideally, a permanent filler should not cause

tissue reactions, be easy to inject, feel natural and be readily removable should the need arise. It should also be totally stable once in position. Unfortunately no filler currently exists which satisfies all these criteria.

Furthermore, doubts have arisen regarding the long-term effects of such fillers. Once injected, the body often forms significant scar tissue around the injected substance making removal extremely difficult without producing noticeable scarring. In addition, many permanent fillers have a tendency to form hard lumps over time. Even if the filler remains soft, over a long period of time there is a chance of it migrating slowly to an undesirable position. If a defect has been overcorrected – i.e. the amount of permanent filler injected is too great – it cannot be rectified easily and will remain overcorrected.

It is thus easy to understand why permanent fillers are not popular with most practitioners, and in general we do not recommend their use for treating soft-tissue defects. However, they are useful when placed next to bone to treat contour irregularities or asymmetries.

Permanent but Removable Implants

Several materials have been developed to augment areas such as the folds from nose to mouth (naso-labial furrows) and the lips. The commonest product used is e-PTFE (polytetrafluoroethylene), a non-toxic, inert material which is readily accepted by the body and that can be easily removed if necessary. The product is available in solid strips or tubes, which can be inserted (implanted) under the skin. The tubular variety allows tissue to grow into the hollow part (lumen) of the implant.

The operation

A small incision is made at the implantation site under local anaesthetic. The implant is threaded under the skin at the required site using a specially designed instrument. The incision is closed with a rapidly dissolvable stitch.

Postoperative events

Swelling and some discomfort or bruising can occur for a few days. Hardness of the material can be felt after the swelling has subsided, as it is not the same as the natural tissue of the body. Also the body produces a scar capsule around the implant, like it does with any foreign body. Migration of the material can occur and it may protrude through the skin if there is inadequate healing.

Paris Lip

Synthetic injectable fillers, fat as well as implants, can be used to enhance the borders of the lips and give more definition. Younger patients may wish to have more prominent and pouting lips. This technique using temporary fillers and implants to produce this look has been named the 'Paris Lip'. Using local anaesthetic, the filler is injected carefully along the white line where the vermilion of the lip meets the normal skin. Some filler is also put into the two ridges above the lip called the philtrum.

SKIN RESURFACING

Skin resurfacing refers to the technique where the superficial layer of the skin is removed in order to allow the raw skin beneath to heal itself. This results in a smoother skin surface, and minor blemishes and scars are removed. A lot of new collagen is induced to form, effectively rejuvenating the skin.

Removal of the surface layer can be achieved by mechanical removal (dermabrasion), using a chemical to partially dissolve the outer layer of skin (chemical peel), or by vaporising the skin using short pulses of heat energy (laser). All three techniques are used for the same basic reasons, and they generally have the same problems and side effects. Which treatment is actually offered depends on the experience and preferences of the surgeon and patient.

Dermabrasion is performed, for anything but very small areas, in an operating theatre under a local or general anaesthetic. Chemical peeling can be done under sedation and analgesia. Apart from the peeling solutions and cotton buds, no special equipment is necessary. Laser treatment requires a specially prepared room (to avoid dangerous reflections of the laser beam, which can cause blindness) and the laser machine itself, which is often very expensive. Laser treatment is the best way to remove tattoos (see 'Removal of Tattoos', pages 194–195).

For the same depth of treatment, dermabrasion heals more quickly than either chemical peels or laser treatment. Chemical peeling (in skilled hands) may be more suitable for dark skin. Laser treatment works well on thread veins (see pages 189–193). Dermabrasion is a difficult technique to learn and requires surgical skill, whereas laser treatment is easy to do once the machine has been properly calibrated and pre-set. Dermabrasion, done freehand with a power tool, is very flexible in that the surgeon can vary the depth of treatment to remove small scars and blemishes.

For all three treatments, if the practitioner is over ambitious and tries to treat the skin too deeply, there is a risk of disfiguring scarring. It is necessary therefore to err on the side of caution and aim for the improvement rather than total eradication of any skin blemishes.

During the healing phase after any of these treatments, all the various cell types in the skin have to grow and multiply. If the skin is exposed to bright light during this time the pigment cells are likely to be over stimulated resulting in brown patches. Often patients never expose the treated skin to strong sunlight, having been told by their surgeon that sun damage was the main cause of their problem in the first place. This results in the treated area remaining paler and less weathered than the surrounding area.

Dermabrasion

Dermabrasion or the 'sanding' of the skin is a procedure used in selected cases and sites to remove irregularities in the skin surface. It is used in young people to treat acne scarring and it is very effective for the treatment of radial lip lines (vertical creases around the lips).

Its benefit was discovered somewhat accidentally from the operation of skin grafting for burns. If a skin graft is taken much too thinly the actual graft isn't much use, but the donor site tended to look a lot better! Surgeons investigated the methods of removing a very thin layer from the skin surface and found that abrasive methods such as wet and dry sandpaper worked well. Nowadays dermabrasion is performed by using a rotating wire brush or diamond wheel to plane down the irregular area. The smooth, even surface that results produces an improved appearance.

Old acne scars and chicken pox marks can be improved as well as certain superficial skin discolorations. Dermabrasion is also used to treat fine lines and wrinkles, especially those in the upper and lower lip regions and around the eyes. It must be emphasised that in severe acne scarring several procedures will be necessary over a period of time.

Preoperative preparation

If you are prone to cold sores you will usually be prescribed a course of anti-cold sore (herpes) medication. The medication is commenced the day before treatment and continued for five days. This is because a herpes infection of the dermabraded skin can lead to scarring, which may require further treatment at a later date.

The operation

You are admitted on the morning of surgery. Small areas can be treated under local anaesthesia. Large areas are best treated under general anaesthesia. The usual technique is to use a small wire brush about 2.5cm (1in) in diameter with a dental drill. The rapidly rotating brush is passed over the skin, producing a superficial graze. The surgeon can vary the depth of the graze until the skin is uniform, bearing in mind that it is important not to go too deep.

At the end of the procedure the treated area will be red and bleeding. A clear plastic sticky sheet like cling film is applied. This prevents scabbing and promotes rapid healing. The patient is discharged home with detailed instructions for postoperative care.

Postoperative events

The abraded area will seep fluid and the general appearance of the treated area is unsightly for a few days. The surgeon will prepare the patient for this beforehand in order to avoid unnecessary anxiety.

Swelling This invariably occurs in the immediate postoperative period. Keeping the head elevated helps to reduce this problem.

Fever This can occur immediately after the procedure. Medication is not often required.

Discomfort Dermabrasion is not nearly as painful as it sounds or looks! It typically feels like a mild sunburn. Any pain that does occur can usually be treated successfully with simple analgesia such as paracetamol.

Itching Sometimes the abraded skin feels very itchy. It is not a good idea to scratch it. Cool air from a fan can be very relieving. Antihistamine tablets can also be helpful.

Insomnia Because of the discomfort sometimes experienced, patients can find it difficult to sleep for a few nights afterwards. Sleeping tablets are prescribed if there is a problem.

Milia Tiny firm white bumps in the skin can appear from three to four weeks post operatively. They may require removal by the surgeon, using the tip of a sharp needle. Sometimes this can be achieved with a rough flannel.

Pigment Changes Pigment alteration will occur in all patients for several weeks. Initially the abraded area will be red, then it will lighten to pink. It may take up to 12 weeks to regain normal pigmentation. Final pigment adjustment may take several months.

Excessive pigmentation (brown patches) is seen in about 10 per cent of cases. It is usually temporary, but can last several months. It must also be emphasised that permanent, excessive or decreased pigmentation can result, but this is rare.

It is extremely important to remember that exposure to sunlight within six to eight weeks following treatment may result in unfavourable discolouration. All patients are strongly urged to stay out of the sun for this length of time and use emollient sun block cream if exposed to sunlight. Sometimes sitting by a window, such as in a car, can be enough to produce brown patches.

Scarring Unfavourable healing is rare but can occur, particularly if a deep abrasion is performed. Thickened (keloid) scarring can occur and mar the result. Further treatment with steroid injections or even a further dermabrasion will be necessary.

Postoperative management

Without doubt dermabrasion can be extremely difficult for a patient postoperatively. Most patients wish to stay out of the limelight until healing has occurred, or until such time as make-up can be applied to hide the initial effects.

It is recommended that patients sleep with their head and torso raised for the first few days to help reduce the swelling.

After one week the cling-film dressing can be removed and the treated area can be patted dry with a clean towel. Sometimes, if the dermabrasion has not been very deep, the skin will stay dry and make-up, including sun block, can be applied at once.

Any prescribed ointments should be applied meticulously as directed by the surgeon. After a few days the face can be washed three times daily with a soft cloth and lukewarm water. Pinkness, dryness and itching can be reduced with a mild anti-inflammatory lotion or cream.

It is important to avoid excessive straining, lifting, bending, intense sunlight or extremes of temperature or strong winds for six weeks. In addition it is vitally important to avoid contact with persons who have herpes simplex (fever blister or cold sores), shingles or chickenpox, impetigo or any other contagious skin disease.

Results
The result of a successful dermabrasion can be extremely pleasing, especially if the original blemish was very noticeable. Despite the initial unpleasant appearance, after the first 24 to 48 hours, patients tend to cope very well. A smooth, pink skin results, which gradually returns to normal colour in the next six to eight weeks. As the aim of treatment is improvement rather than total eradication of all the blemishes, the most common complaint after dermabrasion is that a few blemishes remain. The procedure can be repeated if necessary when the skin has returned to its normal colour.

Chemical Peeling Chemabrasion
Some chemicals, such as strong acids, are corrosive to the skin. Unfortunately, the majority of these chemicals are completely uncontrollable and are not used for therapeutic purposes. However, there are a few chemicals that are deactivated after they have penetrated the skin's surface and they can be used to dissolve the surface layer. These have been used for many years to improve the appearance of the facial skin. There are now several types of peeling agents available that produce excellent results with a rapid recovery time.

The procedure consists of carefully applying a solution containing the corrosive chemical. Usually cotton buds or small swabs are used. The superficial layers of the skin are then dissolved or burnt away in a controlled manner. After a time, which is longer for deep peels, but is generally only a few minutes, the dissolved skin is washed away. Some peeling solutions contain dye to enable the operator to apply it evenly.

Deep peels are usually done after a period of preparation of the skin with tretinoin (vitamin A) and hydrocortisone (steroid) for several weeks. This deepens the peel and makes it more effective. Immediately before any peeling solution is applied, the skin is carefully washed and degreased.

Simple classification of skin peels is based on the depth they penetrate the skin.

Superficial peels
These include glycolic acid, salicylic acid, Jessner's solution (Resorcinol, salicylic acid, lactic acid, ethanol) and 10 per cent Trichloroacetic acid (TCA). These peels are used to treat mild sun damage, acne scars and melasma (brown patches). A course of six to eight treatments is often

required initially to give the skin a more improved appearance. Maintenance sessions are required every three months for best results. These peels are safe with very few side effects. The skin will be red for a few days and recovery is very rapid.

Medium peels

These include strong Jessner's solution, Resorcinol, 15–20 per cent TCA, low concentration phenol. This depth of peel is used to treat fine lines, wrinkles, mild sun damage, superficial scars, and pigmentation. The skin flakes, and there is a recovery period of several days. Side effects include prolonged redness and increased pigmentation.

Deep peels

These include phenol, 30 per cent TCA. These peels have mostly been replaced by laser treatment, and are rarely used in the UK. They are used to treat deeper lines and advanced sun damage. There is a two- to three-week recovery time. Persistent redness, pigmentation and scarring are possible side effects.

It is extremely important to emphasise that for best results, skin protection and a good skin maintenance programme should be followed. A course of anti-cold-sore medication is prescribed as with dermabrasion.

Additional considerations and events for deep peels

Crusting, tightness and redness This will last for at least 10 to 14 days. Frequently, pink discolouration will last three to four weeks. Although a deep chemical peel is not a surgical procedure it can be quite uncomfortable for several days, particularly when the entire face is treated at one time.

Temporary heart problems These have been caused by the application of strong phenol concentrations. The procedure thus needs to be done in a clinic or hospital, where treatment for this problem is available.

Increased or decreased pigmentation Changes in skin pigmentation may occur and may be permanent. The tendency to develop increased skin pigmentation may be increased if you are exposed to sunlight, are taking oral contraceptives or hormone replacement therapy, or become pregnant within six months of treatment. People who have dark skin are more prone to getting pigmentation problems. Exposure to sunlight within six to eight weeks following treatment may result in unfavourable discolouration (as with dermabrasion).

Difference in texture   It is important to realise that the peeled skin will be different in colour and texture from the non-peeled areas and this effect can be permanent.

Thickened scars   These may occasionally occur and require further treatment with steroid injections.

Milia   These little white lumps in the skin can occur as with dermabrasion and are treated along similar lines (see above).

The results of chemabrasion
The subsequent healing that occurs after the superficial layer of the skin has been removed produces a more youthful, healthier and smoother looking skin. This technique can improve sun damage, sun or age spots, wrinkles, pitted acne scars, melasma (excess black pigment in the skin) as well as traumatic scarring.

Laser Skin Resurfacing
This is discussed in more detail on pages 119–122.

MUSCLE DENERVATION

Botulinum Toxin (Botox®)

Botulinum toxin (Botox®) is one of the most toxic substances known to man and is produced by the bacterium *Clostridium Botulinum*. The toxin is extracted from bacteria cultured (grown) in the laboratory. Dried toxin is dispensed in vials as a sterile powder for human use. Saline (salt solution) is added to the vial to reconstitute the dried toxin before it can be injected.

Botulinum toxin relaxes muscle (prevents it contracting) by blocking transmission of the nerve impulse to the muscle. It can take several days to act once injected directly into the muscle and the effect usually lasts for three to four months.

Botulinum toxin has been used in medicine for many years to treat a variety of disabling conditions where muscle tone is increased e.g. in cerebral palsy, facial and neck muscle spasms (ticks) and squints. In the early 1990s, Botox® began to be used for treating facial lines and wrinkles. It has proved to be so successful that it is now thought to be the commonest cosmetic procedure performed globally.

Some patients wish to stop all movement of the treated muscles so that all creases disappear, but this is generally considered to be over-treatment. The best result is to produce a good effect on the wrinkles but to still allow the patient's face to express emotion. Total paralysis of the muscles in significant areas produces rather an odd look. If the wrinkles are too advanced for Botox® to work without abolishing all movement then the patient may be better treated by having surgery such as a browlift or facelift. Unwanted effects from Botox® treatment such as inappropriate unintentional paralysis are usually caused by the surgeon or patient being over ambitious.

The safety of Botox®

Although Botox® is one of the most toxic substances known to man it is generally accepted that it is one of the safest cosmetic treatments available. The lethal dose of Botulinum Toxin is 3,000 units whereas the standard dose given to treat forehead, crow's feet and frown lines rarely exceeds 50 units. Side effects are extremely rare and always temporary.

How Botox® works

Dynamic facial wrinkles and unsightly lines of facial expression result from over activity of the underlying facial muscles. By preventing these muscles from contracting, the cause of the wrinkle is eliminated and in time the wrinkle becomes less prominent and can even disappear completely. It must be stressed that lines caused by aging and sun damage will not respond to Botox®. This method of treating facial wrinkles is known as the 'hibernation treatment' because the muscle 'goes to sleep' or is in hibernation.

Common treatment sites

Botox® is used to treat the following areas of lines and wrinkles on the face:

- Horizontal forehead lines and wrinkles
- Vertical lines and folds between the eyebrows (glabellar lines)
- Crows feet (outer margins of the eyelids) and horizontal lines in the lower eyelids
- Turkey neck and horizontal necklines
- Downturned corners of the mouth
- Chin puckering

The procedure

The benefits of Botox® treatment are operator-dependent. In other words, the skill of the person doing the injecting influences the results. It is important that the practitioner has a good knowledge of facial anatomy so that only the muscles that are producing the unwanted wrinkles are affected.

The injections take only a few minutes to administer. Only the very finest needles are used so that injection pain should be minimal. In some cases a topical local anaesthetic cream is used to numb the skin. The appropriate muscles are injected at strategic points on the face and forehead using a very fine needle. Ice packs can be applied afterwards to reduce swelling.

Duration of action

This varies from patient to patient. In general the effects from the initial injections should last from three to four months. Having regular injections as soon as the muscles regain their activity will cause them to gradually shrink in size. The result is that the intervals between injections can become longer in many patients. Some of our patients come for only two injections per year. If injections are given too frequently, usually more frequently than every two months, a resistance can develop rendering treatment ineffective.

The side effects of Botox®

Redness Redness over the injection sites can last for a few hours. Occasionally an area of bruising can develop if an underlying vein has been accidentally punctured.

Generalised reactions These can occasionally occur. They include nausea, fatigue, flu-like symptoms, headaches and skin rashes (very rare).

Drooping of upper eyelid This can sometimes occur if the injected toxin migrates through the surrounding tissues to affect the muscle that elevates the eyelid. This effect is temporary and can be readily reversed with eye drops.

Drooping of the eyebrow This can occasionally occur if the forehead muscle becomes too weak after injection and droops. The effect will spontaneously reverse in the fullness of time.

Drooping of the lower eyelid This can occasionally occur after injecting the crow's feet area.

Asymmetry of facial expression This can occur, but is only temporary.

Resistance A patient can develop a resistance whereby she no longer responds to the effect of injected Botox®.

Allergic reactions These can occur, but rarely.

Recommended post injection instructions

It is not advisable to touch, rub or massage the treated area for at least three to four hours afterwards in order to prevent the Botox® from migrating into adjacent tissues or muscles, which may precipitate an unwanted side effect.

Patients should stay upright for a few hours and certainly not lie down for four hours afterwards. Some authorities recommend repeatedly tensing treated muscle groups for three to four hours afterwards as the toxin works better in active muscles.

Other uses of Botox®

Excessive sweating (hyperhydrosis) Excessive sweating or hyperhydrosis occurs in about one per cent of the population and is thought to be of genetic origin. It is caused by over activity of one type of sweat gland (the eccrine gland). These glands are found throughout the body but are concentrated on the palms of the hands, soles of the feet and in the armpits. When injected into the skin of the armpit, Botox® blocks the action of the nerves that supply the sweat glands thereby preventing them from producing sweat. The effect lasts from four to seven months.

Change of facial proportions Botox® is increasingly being used to reduce the width of a wide jawline if the excessive width is due to over-development of the jaw muscles. Large doses are injected into the powerful muscles used in chewing, causing them to reduce in volume. The results are usually permanent.

Migraine Botox® has shown to be successful in treating some patients who suffer from regular attacks of migraine. The mechanism of action is unclear and research is ongoing.

Contraindications to Botox® injections

Botox® injections are contraindicated in the following circumstances:

- Known allergy to Botox® or previous problems with Botox®
- Pregnancy and breast-feeding
- Known muscle diseases or taking drugs used to relax muscles

COSMETIC LASER SURGERY

The word laser is an abbreviated term for Light Amplification by Stimulated Emission of Radiation. A laser is a device that produces a powerful, controlled beam of energy (usually in short bursts or pulses). This beam is made of light particles called photons of one particular colour or wavelength. When this powerful light beam strikes its specific target, it generates thermal (heat) energy, which produces its desired effect.

The last few years have seen the development of an assortment of lasers that have a variety of clinical applications in cosmetic surgery as well as in other branches of medicine. In some situations, lasers have superseded previously established treatments.

Laser technology is constantly being developed and upgraded in the field of cosmetic surgery in an attempt to satisfy public demand for improved aesthetic results with the minimum of inconvenience, discomfort and recovery time.

Lasers Commonly Used Today

Ruby laser

The Ruby laser is particularly useful in the removal of tattoos (see page 195) and pigmented skin lesions e.g. brown birthmarks and freckles. Usually no anaesthesia is required and the sensation is similar to an elastic band being flicked onto the skin. A mild rash occurs for a few days afterwards.

Yag laser

The commonest use of this laser is in the removal of tattoos and brown skin lesions e.g. freckles. In removing tattoos various lasers are used to remove the different colours usually associated with modern tattoos. The Yag laser is useful in removing black and red pigment but poor at some green pigments, which respond better to the Ruby laser.

CO2 laser

One of the commonest uses of CO2 lasers is to resurface facial skin and smooth out lines and wrinkles. This can range from small areas such as upper and lower lips to whole-face resurfacing. It is particularly effective in skin which has been sun damaged. It is very effective in treating fine lines in the lower eyelids and crow's feet at the sides of the eyes.

The ability of CO2 lasers to remove lesions from the skin make them useful in removing small to medium-sized birthmarks, which would otherwise have to be excised (cut out) and possibly grafted in conventional surgery. This excision and subsequent suturing of the skin edges under tension can produce an unfavourable cosmetic result e.g. ectropion (drooping) in the lower eyelid (see page 96). Treatment with a CO2 laser is thus a preferable alternative.

Skin Resurfacing, Removal of Facial Wrinkles

Lasers are successfully used to rejuvenate or resurface skin that has been damaged by the sun, aging or scarring. They can also be used to remove small and medium sized skin blemishes e.g. certain moles and birthmarks.

There are a number of different lasers used for skin resurfacing. The commonest types in use are known as Scanned CO2, Pulsed CO2 and Nd:Yag lasers (see above). These lasers are highly sophisticated examples of advanced technology with a precise and accurate mode of action. This means that a pre-selected depth of skin can be accurately destroyed and removed by controlling the intensity and duration of the laser beam. The damaged skin then heals over the following few days yielding a smoother, rejuvenated looking surface.

Method

Laser resurfacing is performed under local or general anaesthetic depending on the area to be treated and patient/surgeon preference, usually on a day care basis. The surgeon wears special eye protective glasses and the patient's eyes are covered with shields that protect the eyes from serious damage by the laser beam. The technique involves firing a circular pulsed laser beam over adjacent areas on the skin surface to be treated.

Aftercare

The same conditions, sequelae and treatment apply as for dermabrasion and chemical peel (see pages 110–115).

Vascular (Blood Vessel) Lesions (Blemishes)

Vascular lesions suitable for laser treatment are those caused by small, dilated blood vessels near the surface of the skin. These dilated blood vessels may be concentrated over a specific area of skin producing a red/blue area of skin discolouration (Haemangioma, Port Wine Stain) or be scattered and less concentrated or even occurring singly, e.g. Thread (Spider) Veins on the face and legs (see pages 189–193).

The dye laser, which utilises a yellow dye, is commonly used to treat vascular lesions. The principle involves using a pulsed laser beam the energy of which is absorbed by the targeted blood vessels. This destroys the vessels, resulting in a variable amount of bruising. Healing occurs to give an improved skin appearance. Multiple treatments are often necessary to give a favourable result.

Hair Removal

Laser hair removal has become extremely popular in recent years. The hair shaft is heated with the laser pulse. The heat passes down the shaft and destroys the hair follicle. The hair then falls out.

Because hair growth is cyclical, not all hairs in an area will be at the same maturation stage, hence not all follicles in an area will be destroyed at any one time. Several sessions will therefore be required to achieve a satisfactory result. About a quarter to a third of hairs in an area will be removed in any one session. (See 'The Treatment of Hair Loss', pages 200–213.)

Tattoo Removal

Lasers are now used to treat the majority of tattoos in clinical practice. Removing tattoos is a difficult undertaking, and usually requires more than one type of laser to remove all the colours. Black and red are easier to remove than green, yellow and purple. Often, between 10 and 15 treatment sessions are necessary. (See 'Removal of Tattoos', pages 194–195.)

The Future of Laser Treatments

More and more women are seeking a remedy for fine lines, wrinkles and skin laxity which is less invasive, shows minimum if any signs of intervention and requires less or no recovery time. To this effect newer and more sophisticated lasers are being produced. One currently attracting attention is the fractional laser, which treats small areas of skin leaving 'bridges' of untreated skin in between. Preliminary results show a favourable outcome and a speedier healing process with significantly reduced recovery time.

INTENSE PULSED LIGHT (IPL)

Intense pulsed light (IPL) utilises a similar principle to laser technology (see above), but with subtle differences that make it more adaptable and therefore more applicable to certain situations.

The Difference Between IPL and Lasers

A laser starts with pulsed light but eliminates all but one wavelength (or colour) of light. A laser therefore can deliver only one colour (or wavelength) of light at a time. Pulsed light can deliver thousands of colours of light at a time. Pulsed light devices use 'cut off' filters to selectively deliver the desired wavelengths. These wavelengths can be pre-selected to target specific structures on the skin surface e.g. hair, blood vessels, and can be modified with each pulse.

Longer wavelengths penetrate deeper into the skin and avoid damage to the skin surface, whereas shorter wavelengths are used to treat more superficial skin structures and avoid damaging deeper parts of the skin.

IPL can be delivered in pulses or bursts of one to five pulses at a time. The duration of each pulse and the time between pulses can be modified with each treatment site.

Applications

IPL can improve sun damage, fine wrinkles, freckles, pigmentation, large pores, rosacea, brown age spots and dilated capillaries. IPL is also used in hair removal. Treatment usually takes less than an hour and feels like a rubber band snapping on the skin, similar to a laser. Usually the procedure can be performed without any anaesthetic. Although IPL is becoming increasingly popular, it must be realised that it does not remove tattoos, despite claims to the contrary. (See 'Removal of Tattoos', pages 194–195.)

Vascular lesions

The treatment of vascular lesions utilises the same principle as with the dye laser, (see above, page 121). Treatment usually takes a few minutes and no anaesthetic is required. IPL is used to treat spider veins in the face and legs as well as rosacea. Normal activities can be resumed the following day. The skin will become pink for a while and it takes several months to achieve the full beneficial effects.

Hair removal

IPL is now becoming one of the commonest methods used for hair removal. (See also above, page 121, and 'The Treatment of Hair Loss', pages 200–213.) The pulsed light is absorbed by the hair follicles, which are damaged and subsequently fail to produce new hairs.

The fair-skinned, dark-haired individual is the ideal candidate for treatment although more modern machines are being developed which can treat most skin types.

A gel is applied to the skin. A hand held unit is then placed over the area covered by the gel and a series of pulses of light is fired over the skin. This destroys the hair follicles and when the gel is removed, much of the hair is removed with it. The remaining hair in the treated areas usually falls out within two weeks.

Because of the number of different phases of the hair growth cycle (see pages 206–207), about five or six treatments are necessary to obtain a favourable result. Results are not permanent and further treatments will be required in the future.

A suntan must be avoided wherever possible prior to treatment as on rare occasions the machine can cause an accidental burn by mistaking the brown pigment in the skin for that in the hair or spider vein. For the same reason, all make-up must be removed prior to treatment.

Skin rejuvenation

IPL works without breaching the skin surface, unlike the case with resurfacing caused by high energy pulsed CO_2 and Erbium YAG lasers. It treats the damaged superficial layer of the skin, while delivering thermal energy to the deeper tissue, resulting in a firmer, tighter skin.

With a special handpiece, pulses of light are delivered to the skin, which stimulates new collagen production, removes pigment and blood vessel changes, thereby rejuvenating the skin. This method is more suitable for patients with only minor signs of aging. It is most commonly used in the face, neck, chest and back of hands.

The skin will appear flushed initially, and capillaries and age spots may become more visible initially, before the appearance starts to improve.

RADIOFREQUENCY SKIN REJUVENATION

Radiothermoplasty

Capacitive Radiofrequency (CRF) technology was introduced in the UK in 2004 as a treatment for skin rejuvenation. It has been used for several years in the USA with some degree of success.

It is a safe, non-invasive, no-recovery-time single treatment, which tightens and contours skin, improving its tone and texture by contracting collagen fibres and stimulating new collagen growth in the area of skin that has been treated. It works well on all skin types and works on the entire face and neck.

Mode of action

When the collagen present in all the skin layers deteriorates as a result of aging, sun damage or hereditary factors, the face begins to sag and wrinkle. CRF technology safely heats the skin layers to shrink or tighten collagen fibres and stimulates new collagen growth. The tightening effect is usually noticed immediately after treatment, with improved skin tone and texture. The new collagen growth continues for the next four to six months further enhancing the initial results.

The procedure

The procedure is performed in a doctor's office or surgery as a 'lunchtime procedure'. Usually no anaesthetic is required, but local anaesthetic cream or nerve blocks can be used if you are nervous or have a low pain threshold.

The area to be treated is drawn on the skin. The practitioner applies the handpiece on the skin and the energy is applied in short bursts. With each burst of energy, you will experience a brief heating sensation. The skin is cooled before, during and immediately after each burst of energy to protect it and make it more comfortable.

Depending on the size and site of the area to be treated, the duration of the procedure varies from 20 minutes to two hours. Afterwards the patient can go home and resume normal activities. There is no special aftercare regime but it is recommended to follow a good skin-care programme.

Temporary redness of the skin and a minor degree of swelling may occur afterwards but this normally resolves within 24 hours. Occasional blisters and skin irregularities have been reported. Depending on the initial skin appearance and condition, results can last for a few years when a repeat procedure can be performed.

Conclusion

As invasive cosmetic surgeons, we do not routinely offer this procedure, primarily because, in our opinion, the results fall far below the standard we would normally expect from surgery. Indeed, the manufacturers of this device state quite clearly that results are limited and should only be offered to those with minimal signs of aging and who do not have loose, hanging skin on the face and who do not wish to have invasive surgery.

Nevertheless, testimonials from satisfied patients clearly demonstrate that there is a place for this procedure. No doubt with improved technology, results will also improve and, who knows, one day we may end up performing this procedure instead of the invasive but highly successful surgery we perform today.

Correction of Protruding Ears

O toplasty is the name given to the procedure used to 'pin back' protruding ears. This condition is inherited and can cause significant embarrassment because of the prejudice that exists against it. It is possible for girls especially to hide their ears with their hair, but they might come to dread windy days or going swimming.

In all people the ears are not completely symmetrical and it is normal for one ear to stick out further than the other. The ears are considered to be abnormally protruding if the distance between the side of the head and the outermost part of the ear is more than 20mm (¾in). The aim of surgery is to reduce this distance to about 15mm (½in), well within the normal range. It is not normal to have the ears tight against the side of the head, even though patients do occasionally request this. Usually the upper part of the ear projects more than the lower. The shape of the ears does not seem to affect hearing in any way.

The medical name for the ear flap is the pinna, and so this operation is also called a pinnaplasty. The pinna has two parts: the inner part – the concha (from the Latin meaning 'shell') – is funnel-shaped and leads into the ear canal; the outer part – the helix – spirals round the concha. There is a tight fold between the two so the helix often protrudes less than the concha.

There are two ways in which the ears can protrude more than usual. The concha might be unusually long or large, or the angle between the concha and the helix might not be properly formed so the helix extends sideways rather than going backwards, the usual position. Often both conditions exist in severe cases. Otoplasty can reduce the size and projection of the concha if it is too big and establish the normal angle between the concha and the helix. It is not usually possible to reduce the size of very large ears that have a normal shape. This is because of the complex shape of the ear. If a part is removed, the resulting defect tends to be visible. However, oversized earlobes can be reduced quite easily.

The ear shape fully develops early in childhood and surgery can be performed as early as the fifth year of life to avoid classroom teasing. Children can be very cruel if they note an abnormality such as jug ears and victims can be bullied and psychologically harmed. This can also cause heartache to parents.

The operation can be easier to perform when the cartilages are soft and thin and more pliant, as in children. In severe cases it may sometimes not be possible to achieve an entirely normal appearance.

The operation

The patient is admitted on the morning of surgery. A general anaesthetic is given to young children whereas local anaesthesia and sedation may be preferred in older children and adults. Local anaesthetic and adrenaline are injected into the operation sites on the backs of the ears.

The incision is made in the groove behind the ear so that scars are hidden from view. The skin over the back of the ear is lifted away from the cartilage. If the concha is too large, a strip of cartilage is taken from the lateral (outer) part and a row of sutures is placed to bring the lateral (outer) edge of the concha closer to the head. The cartilage between the concha and the helix is then bent round to form the normal fold and secured with another row of sutures. The skin is then re-draped and any excess skin is removed. The skin is usually stitched with dissolvable sutures.

At the end of the procedure a turban bandage is usually applied for 24 hours and removed before discharge home the following day. If the operation is performed as a day case the patient can remove the bandage themselves the following day. Thereafter a bandage is worn at night until healing is complete, which takes about six weeks.

Postoperative events

The usual immediate result is that the ears are bruised and swollen and over corrected. The ears come out to a normal position after a few days.

Bruising and swelling This is inevitable, and will usually resolve after about two weeks. If blood collects under the skin forming a lump called a haematoma (see page 39), it may have to be removed. If a significant haematoma is left untreated it can distort the ear cartilage or produce bad scarring of the skin, either of which could produce a very bad result. The typical 'rugby-player' or 'cauliflower' ears are caused by recurrent injuries resulting in bleeding under the skin.

Pain and discomfort This will be variable and medication is only required during the first 24 to 48 hours postoperatively. The ears can be very tender for a few days.

Scars Usually the incision is hidden in the fold at the back of the ear and is unlikely to be obvious. However, in those cases where a significant abnormality of the ear has been corrected it is sometimes necessary to place an incision, and therefore produce a scar, on the outside of the ear where it might be visible.

Infection Infections can sometimes occur and require antibiotic treatment. Rarely the wound may require to be resutured if a severe infection has caused the skin edges to come apart.

Inadequate correction or recurrence of the problem Sometimes the final position of the ears may prove unsatisfactory and a further procedure may be required. This is more likely in cases of severe deformity or where the ear cartilages are very strong. Recurrence usually occurs in the upper part of the ears and it may be necessary to resuture the cartilage at a revision procedure.

The two rows of sutures hold the ear cartilage in its new position while healing and scar formation make the shape permanent. If the ears are pulled sharply soon after the operation the stitches in the cartilage will pull out and the ears will go back to their original shape. This is unlikely to happen during the daytime because the ears are so tender – thus you are not likely to yank them in any way! – but it can happen while you are asleep, turning over on the pillow. This is why it is necessary to protect the ears at night by applying a bandage around the head during the postoperative phase.

The ears can protrude again if dissolvable sutures are used in the cartilage. When the sutures dissolve the cartilages might still have enough spring left to resume their old shape. In order to avoid this possibility many surgeons use permanent sutures in the cartilage.

Permanent sutures can themselves cause problems, however; they might become visible as lumps or the ends can even poke through the skin. If many months have elapsed since the operation these permanent sutures will have done their job by then and can be easily removed under local anaesthetic as a day care procedure. This added procedure doesn't detract from the success of the operation. In any event, the need to remove these sutures is unusual.

Abnormal appearance Surgeons find it easiest to control the middle part of the ears. Sometimes the upper and lower parts of the ears come to lie further out than the middle. This is called the 'telephone ear' deformity. It can be corrected by inserting more sutures as required. If the cartilages are strong and the skin is thin sometimes the reconstructed fold between the concha and the helix becomes visible as a very sharp ridge giving an 'operated-on' appearance. Again, it is usually possible to correct this by revision surgery.

Asymmetry It should be stressed that both ears are never exactly alike even in the normal state. Perfect symmetry is thus not a reasonable expectation.

Skin loss On rare occasions a small area of skin covering the ear may be lost as a result of impaired circulation caused by bruising or infection. A tidy-up procedure may occasionally be necessary to achieve the best results.

Result

After the operation the ears that used to be a source of great embarrassment should look normal. This gives you the freedom to choose any hairstyle you like and means that you no longer have to worry about hiding them. Otoplasty is one of the most frequent and successful operations in cosmetic surgery, and the result is permanent.

Reshaping the Nose

Corrective nasal surgery, or rhinoplasty, is one of the commonest cosmetic procedures performed today. It is carried out by Ear Nose and Throat (ENT), Maxillofacial and cosmetic surgeons.

The operation is performed to repair injuries that have caused a noticeable deformity, and also when the nose has become an unacceptable shape during ordinary growth and development. The modern operation dates from the middle of the 19th century and the pioneering work of Jacques Joseph in Germany. Many of his techniques and even his instruments are still in use today.

The structure of the nose is analogous to a marquee, in which the canvas (the skin) is draped over and supported by a framework of poles or supporting beams (the nasal bones and cartilages). The skin is not the same thickness all over – it is quite thin over the bones and much thicker over the tip. The cartilages of the nose tip are springy and prevent the nostrils being sucked inwards on taking a deep breath.

Essentially the nasal contour is changed by removing, shifting or altering the underlying bony and cartilaginous structures. Except in special circumstances (see 'scars', page 135) the operation is performed from inside the nose leaving no external scars.

When a nose is made smaller – the usual operation – it is the inside of the nose (the airway) that is reduced. If a person has some airway obstruction before the operation it tends to be worse afterwards because of the reduction of the air space. The inside of the nose has a number of complex folds that enable it do its job, namely to warm and humidify the inspired air and to direct the airflow towards the smell-sensitive parts on sniffing. Sometimes rhinoplasty can interfere with the function of the inside, although usually a surgeon would take a pre-existing obstruction into account and try to open up the airway as part of the operation where possible.

In Afro-Caribbean and Oriental noses, the bones are often flat. Corrective procedures in these cases will usually require an implant placed along the top of the bridge to make them look slimmer and more defined and to improve the profile. The nostrils may need to be reduced as well.

At the preoperative consultation, the shape of the new nose is carefully discussed with the patient. There are significant limitations to how much can be achieved, because the skin has to redrape around its new underlying framework. The nature of the skin can have an important effect on the result obtainable. In patients who have thick skin, which is often greasy, the skin does not retract very well. If the frame of the nose is reduced too much in those cases there will be an ugly excess of skin characterised by a bulbous tip that droops. In those patients who have very thin skin, every asymmetry or irregularity of the bones and cartilages can be rendered visible.

The skin tends to get even thicker after the operation in those who had thick skin before, especially where the skin is thickest at the tip. After rhinoplasty, thickened tip skin can take several years to settle. Some patients have strong cartilages that offer good support to the overlying skin, whereas others have weak cartilages (and thick skin), which make it difficult for the surgeon to achieve a good result. The operation causes scarring beneath the skin overlying the tip, which can further compound these difficulties.

The operation itself can be carried out to a very high degree of accuracy by a competent surgeon, but unfortunately the postoperative swelling and scarring is more unpredictable. This means that it would be most unwise for a surgeon to try to guarantee to you exactly what your nose is going to look like after the operation. In any case the appearance will change with time, rapidly for the first few months but more slowly later on.

We therefore do not recommend or believe in using computerised imaging technology at the preoperative consultation because human tissues cannot be accurately sculpted or refined in the same manner as a piece of metal or wood. Such predicted computer images can easily give you false hopes and unrealistic expectations. The best candidates are those patients who don't like their noses, and who may be very self-conscious of being seen in profile, but who will accept an improvement, even if the new nose isn't perfect.

Normal noses change in shape during life. The shape of the nose of a 60 year old is usually quite different from that of a young person. It is even harder to predict the result of a secondary or revision rhinoplasty; many surgeons are unwilling to undertake revision operations.

The operation

You will be admitted on the morning of the operation. Preoperative photographs are taken. A general or twilight anaesthetic is given (see 'Anaesthesia', pages 60–63). Local anaesthetic and adrenaline are injected under the skin. The nose is packed with material soaked in drugs e.g. cocaine to reduce bleeding and pain.

There are two approaches currently in use, called the open and closed techniques. In the closed technique an incision is made inside the nostrils on each side and the skin is lifted away from the supporting frame. In the open technique an incision is made across the columella (the part between the nostrils). Then the part of the columella in front of the incision is lifted forwards and the skin that covers the tip is undermined. This results in much better exposure of the skeletal structures and is commonly employed in revision surgery or where reconstruction using cartilage grafts is contemplated. This results in a small, hopefully inconspicuous, scar across the columella.

If the patient has a bony hump that needs to be reduced the bones are rasped with a file or the hump is removed with a hammer and chisel, depending on the amount of bone to be removed. Removal of the hump results in the two nasal bones not meeting in the middle, so an incision is made in each bone where it meets the face and the bones are fractured inwards so that each bone again touches its partner in the midline. The tip cartilages are then carefully trimmed to give the desired tip shape. It is important not to remove too much cartilage from the tip, because if they are weakened too much the nostrils will collapse inwards on breathing. Sometimes small pieces of cartilage are taken from the nasal septum (the midline cartilage partition inside the nose which divides it into two halves) or one of the patient's ears and placed as little grafts to aid the tip support and projection. In many cases the nasal septum needs to be trimmed to allow the columella to be lifted.

When the surgeon is satisfied that the result of the operation is the best obtainable he will carefully suture the incisions previously made inside the nose. In nearly every case the nose will then be packed with sterile gauze. This holds the airway open, enables the lining of the nose to adhere to its previous position and reduces postoperative bleeding. The pack is generally removed the following morning.

At the completion of the operation a splint is placed on the nose and secured in position with sticky tape. The splint is removed after seven to 10 days. The purpose of the splint is to immobilise the fractured nasal bones and reconstructed cartilaginous framework so that they heal together in the desired position. It also controls and reduces the swelling and protects the nose from further trauma.

Immediately after the operation the nose is quite vulnerable and without the splint even a slight knock could ruin the result. Nasal fractures heal very quickly and after 10 days or so it would take a significant blow to do any harm. The nose will be as strong as it ever was at about three months, and after six months would be even stronger because the fractured bones once healed are stronger than they were originally. It is very hard to break a boxer's nose again once it has been broken a few times!

The duration of the stay in the clinic is usually no longer than one day. The patient goes home having had the pack removed, but wearing the splint.

Postoperative events

Bruising and swelling Bruising and swelling of the nose and around the eyes occurs in nearly all patients. Most of the bruising and swelling around the eyes subsides within seven days. Slight swelling in the nose that is not generally apparent to the onlooker, but that can be noticed by the patient, may take many months to subside.

Infection and bleeding These may occur as with any operation. Some patients bleed or discharge bloody fluid from the nose for a few days. If the bleeding is more than a slight trickle you must inform your surgeon. Fortunately these complications are uncommon and do not generally give any cause for concern.

Nasal blockage As the tissues inside the nose are swollen afterwards it is not uncommon to experience a variable degree of impairment to breathing. This symptom however usually resolves itself a short time after the operation. It is rare to experience permanent nasal obstruction if it was not already present before surgery. However, many hay-fever sufferers get more allergic symptoms after rhinoplasty and may need stronger treatment than they needed before. Some patients get a feeling of congestion in the sinus at the top of the nose.

Numbness of the tip Numbness in the tip of the nose sometimes occurs and may be present for some weeks after the operation. It usually resolves completely.

Pain and discomfort   Despite the nature of the operation, pain and discomfort are surprisingly rare. Painkillers are given as required, but most people don't need them.

Polly beak deformity   Excessive thickening of the skin just above the tip of the nose after the operation is called polly beak deformity. It generally responds to tiny injections of steroid, but may need revision surgery. Skin type is one of the most important factors that determine how pleasing the shape is after the operation. Thin skin will redrape more readily around the newly reconstructed scaffolding of bone and cartilage of the nose. Thick skin will not redrape with the same finesse and having thick skin increases the chance of getting this supra-tip thickening.

Irregularities and asymmetry   Sometimes during the prolonged recovery after rhinoplasty, lumps and irregularities appear when the swelling declines. Generally these also settle, the process being helped by massage. A few patients however may need to have revision surgery.

Problems with implants and grafts   Implants placed along the dorsum (bridge of the nose) can occasionally become displaced in time, and they also confer a low risk of infection. The little cartilage grafts that some surgeons use can disappear because they can be reabsorbed, or occasionally they increase in size and become lumpy.

The wrong shape   Due to the unpredictable nature of scarring and swelling after the operation, rhinoplasty is not an exact science. The aim of a rhinoplasty is improvement. Perfection would be a fluke. Immediately after the operation many patients feel that the nose has been turned up too much. In these cases the surgeon has probably allowed for the effect of gravity and has slightly over corrected the nose to give a better long-term result.

The result seen immediately after the operation is never the final one, and it usually goes on improving throughout the recovery period. Those patients who end up with a result that they find unsatisfactory, may well have had a communication problem with their surgeon at the preoperative-consultation stage. It is vitally important at the preoperative consultation for the patient and surgeon to agree on the proposed changes. However, an absolutely exact replica of the proposed shape is unlikely.

Scars In the vast majority of cases all work is done on the inside of the nose leaving no external scars. However, after the operation, in all cases there will be a layer of scar tissue beneath the skin. Initially a thin layer of scarring will be formed which will temporarily increase in thickness before it thins out again a few months later. Daily massaging of the nasal skin during the recovery period will help the scar tissue to mature favourably.

Immediately after the splint is removed the nasal skin will, in most cases, be stuck firmly to the underlying structures. Massaging the skin will help it recover the normal skin mobility.

If it is necessary to make the nostrils smaller, an incision is made where the outer side of the nostril adjoins the upper lip. Because this is located in a natural body fold, the scar is practically unnoticeable to the average onlooker.

Many surgeons are now using the technique of open rhinoplasty where the nose is opened up to give the surgeon better access to the anatomical components of the nose. This is usually performed using an inverted V-incision in the columella. The scar is usually unnoticeable.

Headache A few patients report headaches or nasal pain after the operation.

Change in sense of smell or taste This occurs very rarely. It is usually temporary, but very rarely can be permanent.

Postoperative management

After discharge from the clinic and until the splint is removed, you will be advised to rest as much as possible, sleep upright, sneeze through the mouth and avoid blowing your nose.

Ice packs can be applied to the eyes to help reduce bruising and swelling. You should wash your hair carefully until the splint is removed as soaking it with water may dislodge it. Glasses may be worn on top of the splint if this is possible but once it is removed it is advised that glasses should not be allowed to rest on the nose for a few weeks. It is usually necessary to have an optician refit your glasses on your 'new' nose. Glasses should be carefully fitted so that the nose pads rest flat on the skin and don't put pressure on only a small area: If they do, they are likely to cause a dent. Contact lenses can be worn again after a few days.

Should a significant haemorrhage occur from the nose after you have been discharged home it is advised that ice packs are applied to the side of the bleeding. After the first 48 hours, bleeding from the nose is very uncommon. If it does occur you must inform your surgeon immediately. It may be necessary to prescribe antibiotics. If the bleeding doesn't stop readily it is occasionally necessary to pack the nose again.

You should avoid strenuous exercise for four weeks. After that time non-body-contact sports are permitted. Body-contact sports are prohibited for six months.

Surgeons vary in how long they keep the splint in place, and sometimes it is necessary to keep the splint on for longer than usual to control the swelling, or if the nasal bones were unstable at the end of the operation. Most surgeons opt for a period of seven to 10 days. On the appointed day, some surgeons let the patients remove the splint themselves, while others arrange for it to be removed in their outpatient clinic. The immediate result on removing the splint is often disappointing, because where it has been resting on the bones there may be a pinched look and the tip will be swollen. Within a day or two, however, this should have dramatically improved, just leaving the residual swelling that slowly subsides over many months.

Results

Most patients are delighted with the result of their rhinoplasty operation, which is generally very successful in experienced hands. You should be much less self-conscious and be able to be seen from all sides with confidence.

It should be stressed again, however, that there is a limit to the corrective procedures possible or recommended. The surgical goal is improvement and it is usually not possible to create the ultimate perfect shape that you may have had in mind.

Some of the limiting factors in rhinoplasty are the contour and shape of the face; the texture and thickness of the skin; the inclination of the chin, lip and forehead; the depth of the angle between the forehead and the nose; the height of the patient and the healing powers of the tissues. The amount of scar tissue formed under the skin after the operation will also have a major influence on the final shape.

Noses that have been severely injured or those that are markedly crooked are technically difficult to correct and a second procedure may be necessary.

As with facelifts, the operation of rhinoplasty has succeeded in producing its own unique problems as exemplified by some well-known celebrities. An 'over operated nose', i.e. one that has undergone several unsuccessful procedures, can look quite bizarre! We wish to stress, however, that such situations are very rare and a rhinoplasty operation performed by an experienced and able surgeon should not yield such an abnormal cosmetic result. You should therefore not be apprehensive about undergoing this procedure, as the results are usually excellent.

Chin Augmentation

Chin enlargement, or mentoplasty, is performed to rectify a receding or weak chin or in conjunction with a nose reshape operation to achieve a better profile.

The operation

The procedure involves the insertion of an implant, and is usually performed under sedation and local anaesthesia, or general anaesthesia if a rhinoplasty is being performed at the same time. A small incision is made in the mouth in the groove where the lower lip joins the front surface of the jaw in front of the gum of the lower teeth. The operation thus leaves no external scars.

The soft tissue of the front of the chin is separated from the bone and a pocket that exactly fits the proposed implant is made. The implant is then inserted so that it lies against the bone. The lower edge of the implant is level with the lowest part of the point of the chin. The implants are usually made of silastic, a firm silicone plastic, although many other materials have been used, including bone grafts and even coral.

Implants are available in various shapes and sizes. The most usual shape is a crescent, the hollow back of the implant following the same curve as the front of the jaw. The implants have more of a bulge on either the top surface, or the bottom surface if it is upside down. In women the implant is usually placed with the bulge uppermost, whereas in men the implant is placed with the bulge downwards. The idea in women is to preserve the feminine shape of the chin while still pushing it forwards. In men the downward bulge masculinises the profile. In some implants the ends of the crescent are considerably extended so that they lie along the edge of the jawbone and give more width.

The surgeon chooses the most suitable type of implant depending on what you want to achieve. The surgeon ensures that the implant is a snug fit in its pocket, so that it cannot move. If there is any movement the implant has to be attached to the bone in some way. The little wound in the mouth is then sutured with dissolvable sutures. Usually some sort of strapping is applied over the chin to reduce the chance of displacement during the healing phase, and to reduce swelling. The strapping is removed after a few days.

Postoperative events

Great care should be taken in the immediate postoperative period to ensure adequate wound healing. Some surgeons recommend frequent mouthwashes. Chewing should be reduced to a minimum so it is best to eat soft or liquid foods for a few days after the operation. Care should be taken when eating and cleaning the teeth.

Recovery is very swift and the final result should be seen within two or three weeks.

When an implant has been in place, resting on the bone for many months, it creates a little hollow for itself as a result of the pressure it constantly exerts on the underlying bony tissue of the chin. This makes it much less likely to move out of position.

Bruising and swelling These are are usually minimal and transient.

Extrusion of the implant The implant can sometimes come out, generally as a result of infection. If this is going to happen it will probably occur soon after the operation, but can sometimes happen many months later. A further procedure will then be required to re-insert the implant at a later date.

Displacement of the implant This can sometimes occur even if the implant was correctly inserted. Further surgery to replace it in the correct position will be necessary. Usually it takes significant trauma to move a stable implant, such as a direct blow from a fist. Occasionally, however, if you habitually lean your chin on your hand over a prolonged period of time – when reading, for example – then movement may occur.

Infection Infection is uncommon and usually responds to antibiotic treatment. It can lead to extrusion of the implant (see above).

Numbness of the lower lip This is a common temporary occurrence. On very rare occasions it can be permanent.

Result

The improved shape of the chin and the better balance of the face should be permanent once the wound around the implant has fully healed. The implant is quite firm, and once it is stable it should not be possible to tell by feeling along the jaw where the bone ends and the implant begins – the implant should be undetectable.

Other operations

Implants can also be placed on the underside of the chin to make the lower part of the face longer. But these are not very stable unless secured into position in some way and this makes the operation more complicated. They are inserted through an incision in the skin just below the jaw in the midline.

If the chin is too long then a small amount of bone can be removed from the point of the chin, either from the front or underneath. Unfortunately the roots of the teeth and the shape of the jaw itself often limit the amount of bone that can be removed, therefore only fairly minor changes can be achieved by this method. The incision is usually made on the underside of the jaw in the natural crease. If there is any excess skin as a result of the bone removal then it can easily be trimmed leaving a single scar line on the underside of the chin, which is not easily visible.

A receding chin can also be treated by a much more complicated operation called a 'sliding genioplasty'. In this operation the lowest part of the jawbone is separated by making a horizontal cut in the bone and then brought forwards. It is held in position by wires or screws. Maxillofacial surgeons commonly perform this operation. The same principle, only moving the lower part of the jaw backwards, can be used to treat a chin that is too long.

Occasionally patients request that various alterations are made to the actual shape of the chin, such as producing a cleft or making a dimple. It is possible to do this in some cases.

Fillers Nowadays there are more long lasting fillers available and these are increasingly being used to augment chins as well as cheeks (see page 91). The fillers commonly used in chin augmentation are Restylane Sub Q (see pages 104–105), Radiesse® (see page 105) and Bio-Alcamid. A simple injection is all that is required. Occasionally local anaesthetic may be used, although its use is kept to a minimum because it is easier for the surgeon and patient to see the effect of the injection without the swelling caused by the anaesthetic.

Sometimes a patient may be wary of having a permanent filler injected because there is a chance that they may not like the result, and permanent fillers can be very hard, if not impossible, to remove once they are in place.

However, there is a neat way of showing the patient exactly how the filler is going to turn out. It is possible to inject a small volume of saline solution, the same volume as the filler would be, into the proposed site. You can then see exactly what the result would be. The saline solution will only stay for about half an hour or so before it is absorbed into the body. Photographs may be taken while it is still present to give a permanent record of the effect. If you like the effect, then the permanent filler can be injected on a subsequent occasion.

This same technique can be used over the cheekbones to show the effect of a permanent filler there.

This manoeuvre is one of the few examples in cosmetic surgery of where an exact simile of the intended result can be achieved, which is transient and produces no ill effects.

Surgery of the Breasts

BREAST AUGMENTATION (ENLARGEMENT)

Breast enlargement is one of the commonest cosmetic surgical procedures performed in this country today. Despite the silicone breast-implant controversy that blighted this operation in the late 1980s and early 1990s, silicone breast implants are now very firmly back on the agenda.

There are no exercises or medications currently available that can safely, effectively and permanently increase breast size. The current recognised, accepted and regularly performed method for increasing breast size involves the insertion of a silicone breast implant behind the natural breast tissue.

Various other methods have been tried intermittently over the years with limited success, most notably fat injections, which never seemed to gain popularity in the UK because of the high incidence of failure and complications. However, it seems that this method is currently experiencing a resurgence in popularity as some surgeons, especially from the USA, claim consistently good, but rather limited results.

From time to time adverts appear in the press claiming a revolutionary technique to enhance breast size. Usually such claims employ the use of tablets, creams or local stimulation such as vacuum pumps. We urge the reader to exercise extreme caution when considering these options, as invariably these claims are a short-term scam to make huge amounts of money for the perpetrator.

No one should ever purchase any breast-enhancing oral preparations that are advertised in the press unless they have previously discussed it with a qualified medical practitioner. Any medical preparation that has received proper approval for the treatment of any condition will have previously been extensively researched. Results will have been published in the medical press, and, if it is a non-prescription drug, it will be readily available in shops or chemists.

Why Seek Breast Enlargement?

In general, three types of women seek breast enlargement. The first consists of those who have never had a full development of breast tissue and simply wish to become larger.

The second group consists of those who may have had normal breast development but who wish to become larger because their breasts have decreased in size following pregnancy, weight loss, or aging.

The third group consists of those who have suffered previous breast disease, particularly cancer, where breast tissue has been surgically removed. These patients seek breast reconstruction, which usually involves the insertion of a breast implant.

The types of implant available

At the time of publication of this book, all breast implants currently available have an outer silicone plastic shell called silastic, which has either a smooth or textured (rough) surface. It is the nature of the filling substance that differentiates the types of implant that are available. Implants are manufactured in various shapes and sizes to suit different requirements.

Other filling agents besides those described below have been used in the past but have been withdrawn because of safety issues e.g. Trilucent implants (vegetable oil) and Hydrogel implants (salt and sugar solutions).

Standard silicone gel This filling has a long history of reliable use with a natural feel. The main disadvantages are the possibility of leakage and rupture.

Firm cohesive silicone gel This filling is made to a solid consistency that maintains its shape. The gel does not ooze if the implant ruptures. The main disadvantages are its high cost, an unnatural feel and asymmetry with rotation of the implant.

Saline This is a biocompatible filler with a long history of use. The main disadvantages are that they are unsuitable for women with little breast tissue as well as being more prone to wrinkling and rupture. Saline implants come with smooth and textured surfaces and once inserted into the breast pocket can be inflated with saline to the required size. Unfortunately these implants are not very popular with surgeons in the UK as they have an increased tendency to rupture as a result of the friction forces between the saline filler and the silicone shell, or deflate due to failure of the filling valve.

The shape of implants

Over the last 25 years, implant manufacturers have increasingly developed a wider range of sizes, shapes and types of implant. The 'round' implant is the most popular shape used by surgeons in the UK. Some surgeons routinely favour the 'teardrop' or 'anatomical' shape. In addition, round implants come in various forward projections otherwise referred to as the 'profile'. Currently there are low, high and extra high profiles available.

Every woman is unique and the size and shape of the implant is usually determined at the time of consultation although the final decision will be made at the time of the operation.

The surface of implants

The implants commonly available today have two types of surface referred to as smooth and textured. A smooth surface, as its name suggests, consists of a smooth all over silicone shell surface encasing a volume of filler e.g. silicone gel or saline (see above).

A textured implant consists of a rough silicone shell surface. Some manufacturers provide a range of implants with different degrees of roughness or texture. Research papers have clearly shown a reduction of capsular contracture (see below) with the textured variety of implant.

Structural variations in silicone implants

Some silicone gel implants have two silicone shells. The outer shell can be inflated with saline solution to add further volume to the implant.

The whole implant is first inserted into the breast pocket. The required volume of saline is injected through a tube attached to the surface of the outer shell. There is a one-way valve at the point of attachment of the tube to the shell to keep the injected saline in. Once the required volume of fluid has been injected the tube is pulled out leaving the inflated shell at the required volume and guarded by the one-way valve.

Thus it is possible to finely tune the breast size with saline at the time of the operation without having to remove the implant and try out different sizes. It is our opinion that the more physical interference with the breast pocket at operation the more likelihood there is of future severe capsular contracture (see below).

The preoperative consultation

At the preoperative consultation you should have a list of questions for your surgeon in the unlikely event that he will not have covered any of the important points pertinent to this operation. You should ask the following:

1. How big will I be after the operation? We usually tell every patient that it is simply not possible to pick a breast off the shelf, because we can only work with the materials at our disposal, i.e. the patient's tissues. Thus, the amount of breast tissue, covering skin, chest width and patient expectations all influence the size and shape of the implant that it is possible to insert.

   For the patient expecting a larger size than is possible, we tell them that it is impossible to pour a litre of water into a half-litre jug without it spilling over. In other words, there is a limit to how big an implant can be inserted.

   We do not routinely advocate trying out different implants by placing them into a bra. This practice is misleading and can easily lead to disappointment because a bra does not necessarily match the size and elasticity of the breast tissue, nor will it give an accurate assessment of how the breast will look after implantation, bearing in mind that the implant is placed under a mass of tissue.

   With experience, most surgeons will know at preoperative consultation what implant size will be most suitable for each patient. We also do not promise a particular size of breast afterwards because bra sizes do vary according to the manufacturer and it is not always possible to estimate exactly how much the breast will stretch after the implant is inserted. In other words, we can at best only give a patient an approximate idea of the size; making promises can lead to disappointment for patient and surgeon.

   Showing pre- and post-operative photographs is useful, as a patient's reactions will nearly always indicate their likely reaction to the result of the operation.

2. What are the likely complications? Your surgeon should cover each of the points outlined below in detail, especially capsular contracture.

3. How long do the implants last and when should I change them?

4. How long do I need to stay off work?

5. How safe are silicone implants?

6. Any other question you can think of that may be pertinent to your situation if the information is not covered below.

All the main points are covered below and you are advised to familiarise yourself with the facts about breast augmentation beforehand, in order to get the best out of your consultation with your surgeon.

One final point of warning: do not listen to lay counsellors or salespersons (in a commercial clinic) regarding the size. Only an experienced operating surgeon will be able to give you an idea about what size is possible.

The operation

You will be admitted to the hospital or clinic on the morning of the operation. A general anaesthetic is used in most cases, although this procedure is increasingly performed under intravenous sedation and local anaesthesia on a day-care basis in some patients.

The site of the incision (usually about 3–4cm in length) will depend on the surgeon and patient preference. It is most commonly made in the crease underneath the breast. Some surgeons however prefer to make the incision in the armpit or around the areola (the circular pigmented area around the nipple).

A pocket for the implant is created in the breast (see below for more details about the location of the implant). A silicone implant is then inserted into the pocket. The implant may be placed in front of or behind the muscle of the chest. Most surgeons will insert a fine tube drain to let out any fluid that may collect around the implant and this drain is usually removed the following day. The skin is closed with stitches that do not come through the skin surface so that there are no stitch marks. A bandage or supporting bra is usually applied.

The following day before discharge home, the bandage is removed and you will be fitted with a bra. Some surgeons do not advocate wearing tight bras in the immediate postoperative period as they feel it could predispose you to capsular contracture (see below) at a later stage. The sutures may be removed after seven to 10 days.

Location of the implant   Breast implants may be placed in front of or behind the pectoralis (chest) muscle. The location will ultimately depend on the patient as well as the surgeon's preference.

Based on our experience, we prefer to place breast implants in front of the muscle wherever possible, as we consider the results to be superior. However, in patients who have very little breast tissue it is perhaps wiser to place the implant behind the muscle. This is because the chest muscle will give extra padding in front of the implant thereby preventing the implant being felt. If placed in front of the muscle behind a small breast containing only a thin layer of tissue, it is more likely that you will be able to feel the implant through the skin.

Different surgeons have different preferences, and these should be discussed with you at your preoperative consultation.

Postoperative events

Pain and discomfort   This is alleviated with appropriate medication. Most women tell us that the discomfort from this operation is not too severe. Many patients will require at least one opiate injection postoperatively. By the next morning most of the discomfort will have worn off in the majority of patients and they can be discharged home on oral painkillers.

Bleeding and haematoma   On rare occasions, severe bleeding may continue after the operation has been completed, into the pocket created for the implant, resulting in a haematoma (see page 39). The majority of haematomas will occur within a few hours of the operation. Secondary bleeds can occur as late as 10 days after the operation, but this situation is extremely rare and there is usually a predisposing cause. The affected breast will become hard, swollen and extremely tender.

This is a surgical emergency and if you have already been discharged from hospital, you must notify your surgeon immediately. You will need to be taken back into theatre to drain the collection of blood. The implant will be removed and the source of the bleeding will be sought, after all the clots have been evacuated. Any bleeding points are cauterised. Once the surgeon is satisfied that there is no further bleeding the implant is re-inserted and the wound sutured.

Failure to drain an excessive collection of blood in the pocket created for the implant will inevitably lead to a hardening of the breast when the blood has clotted and will invariably result in early capsular contracture (see below).

Infection This uncommon complication may lead to the breakdown of the wound, necessitating the temporary removal of the implant. This will usually occur within the first 10 days after the operation. After the infection has subsided a new implant can safely be reinserted.

Very rarely an insignificant haematoma (see above) may become infected and result in the formation of an abscess (collection of pus). The patient becomes unwell and suffers discomfort. A further surgical procedure to drain the abscess will be required.

Chronic low-grade infection may occur with any surgical implant. Such infection, at any site in the body, may be associated with a number of symptoms including tiredness, weakness, intermittent temperatures, muscle aches and pains. Although this is a very rare occurrence it may account for some of the media reports that accuse silicone of being the direct cause of these symptoms.

Scars Every attempt is made to make scars as short and as inconspicuous as possible. A sagging breast has a natural crease underneath and scars placed there will not normally be noticeable except perhaps when lying down on a topless beach. When there is little skin and breast tissue at the outset there will not be significant breast crease formation after surgery and therefore a scar placed at the lower border of the breast will not be hidden as readily.

Most women consider a short visible scar a small price to pay for an otherwise pleasing result. On rare occasions scars may have to be revised (see 'Improving Unsightly Scars', pages 196–199) if they become stretched or thickened, but in most cases a barely perceptible thin line results.

Capsular contracture Immediately after the operation, the process of healing begins. The body's complex healing system recognises that there is a foreign body (the breast implant) present inside it. The body's immune system treats a breast implant in exactly the same way as any other invader, e.g. a virus or bacterium, and thinks that this invader is trying to harm the body.

The net result is that a 'protective' layer of scar tissue is formed around the implant. This layer of scar tissue effectively seals off or entombs the 'invading implant' from the rest of the body. This protective layer of scar tissue is called a 'capsule'. It is usually formed a few days after the operation and is thin and supple. This is considered a normal occurrence and results in soft, natural feeling breasts.

In some cases however, for reasons that are not yet clearly understood, this capsule can misbehave, usually in one of three ways. It can either contract around the implant, gradually increase in thickness, or both. This process is commonly known as capsular contracture. On some occasions a triggering mechanism can be identified in the form of a recent infection or illness suggesting that an immune response may be directly responsible. A breast infection (mastitis) nearly always produces capsular thickening and contracture. We have also noticed that even a severe psychological event can trigger this response e.g. a family bereavement.

The result is that the breasts can assume differing consistencies in texture, ranging from slightly firm to very hard. In addition the breast may become misshapen. This condition is not usually painful, although discomfort can sometimes occur. Severe pain is extremely rare. It must be further appreciated that this can happen at any time after the operation from weeks to months to years, and occur in one or both breasts. Overall, with modern implants, three to six per cent of women experience unnatural hardening of their breasts.

It must also be stressed that capsular contracture does not imply that something is seriously wrong. Every patient will experience a degree of encapsulation after implantation. The degree and severity of capsular thickening and contracture will determine the consistency of the breasts.

In the majority of cases, capsules do not present a problem to the patient. In cases where there is pain or discomfort or where the breast becomes misshapen, further surgery will be necessary, usually in the form of surgical excision (removal) of the capsule (capsulectomy) or cutting the capsule surgically to release the constricting effect (capsulotomy). It is important to realise that capsular contracture can recur. There are currently no known oral preparations or injections available that will safely reverse or reduce capsular contracture.

Capsular contracture is not a result of improper or inadequately performed surgery, but a combination of intrinsic and extrinsic factors outside the control of the surgeon, which ultimately result in variable hardening of the breast. There is currently no method of determining if a patient is going to be vulnerable to capsular contracture e.g. a blood or skin test.

Breast investigations Concern has been raised about the possibility of achieving accurate results from mammography or ultrasound scanning in the presence of silicone implants. Nowadays breast-screening investigations in patients with silicone implants are commonplace and do not present a problem to the trained radiologist.

Breast lumps   Many women are concerned that breast implants will conceal, or make it impossible to palpate (feel), a breast lump should it ever occur after breast implantation. A breast lump will still be felt by the woman or by the examining doctor because the implant is situated behind the breast. Indeed there is some evidence that breast lumps are, if anything, easier to feel in the presence of an implant. If a woman with breast implants develops cancer they usually present earlier, which improves the prognosis.

Breast feeding   This is still possible after implantation. There is no evidence that babies who have been breast-fed by mothers with silicone breast implants are at increased risk of developing any illness.

Ptosis (drooping of the breast)   Drooping of the breast can benefit from breast augmentation. However, there is a limit to how much an implant can improve ptosis, and augmentation can sometimes make it worse. If the nipple falls below the fold under the breast, concurrent mastopexy (uplift) (see below) is usually advisable. The risks of augmentation alone versus the scarring associated with mastopexy must be especially considered by the patient, her partner and the surgeon.

Wrinkling and folding of implants   These are unpredictable complications that may follow breast implantation. This can become manifest as a result of thin breast tissue, capsular contracture (see above), loss of skin elasticity, very small breasts or excessive weight loss. The result is the appearance of folds or wrinkles on the surface of the breast and may become more obvious when leaning forward without a bra. Wrinkling can also produce little corners on the implant that can sometimes be felt if the overlying breast tissue is too thin. Sometimes it is necessary to insert a different type of implant.

Implant protrusion   Implants can sometimes be felt as a lump in the breast. Although it is possible for the implant to be felt at any site on the breast surface they are most commonly felt at the lower border or sides of the breast particularly when standing upright. Usually they disappear or are less prominent on lying down.

This is due to the fact that the implant stretches the surrounding breast tissue in time, resulting in a thinner layer of tissue surrounding the implant. A point of weakness in this tissue will enable the implant to protrude, especially in the upright position thereby giving the impression that a breast lump is present. This can often give rise to panic but your surgeon will clearly be able to identify this problem and be able to reassure you.

This situation occurs most commonly in women who have had implants placed in front of the muscle and whose breasts were very small in the first instance. The concomitant stretching and thinning of the surrounding breast tissue makes implant protrusion a more likely possibility.

Deflation of the saline implant This occurs due to rupture or failure of the valve in saline implants.

Shape and symmetry It is extremely rare for two breasts to be visibly symmetrical on close scrutiny. With implantation, this asymmetry may be exaggerated further. Sometimes asymmetry may become more apparent after infection (see above), capsular contraction (see above) or deflation of the implant (see above). Where asymmetry is particularly apparent, different size implants may be inserted in an attempt to make the result more symmetrical. Perfect symmetry can never be promised nor guaranteed.

Sensory changes Some impairment of nipple sensation may occur following surgery. This is due to the inevitable damage to the sensory nerves in the breast and nipple areola complex. Nerves may be cut, stretched or damaged at the time of surgery leading to a variety of peculiar sensory changes following surgery.

The nipple and areola can feel totally numb in the immediate postoperative period. This is usually temporary, lasting up to a few days. The area then regains its sensitivity slowly, returning to normal within a few days to a few weeks. Partial sensory loss is only rarely a permanent feature. Total permanent nipple sensory loss is extremely rare. Research has shown that in most women, nipple sensory loss is not an important issue.

More irksome is the sensation of pain or discomfort and extra sensitivity of the nipples. Thankfully this is only a temporary feature in the vast majority of cases.

Sensation in the lower portion of the breast may be impaired until the sensory nerves have recovered. Some patients report temporary 'electric-shock' type sensations in the nipple lasting for a few moments. These usually settle in time.

Leakage of silicone Most modern implants manufactured today have a leak-proof membrane internally, which prevents liquid silicone from leaking or 'bleeding' through the implant shell.

As already stated above, once the implant is in place inside the body, a capsule or layer of scar tissue will form around it. This capsule will act as a further barrier to any liquid silicone that may bleed through the implant shell thereby preventing it from permeating into the surrounding tissues.

Concern has been raised in the past about the possibility that leakage of silicone from breast implants can cause health problems. Actually, the amount of silicone that leaks through the shell of modern implants is extremely small and no health problems have ever been shown to be associated with this.

It is actually quite difficult to avoid silicone in ordinary life as it is a common constituent of food packaging and is found in many cleaning agents. It is very widely used in medicine, in silicone tubing, artificial joints, cardiac pacemakers and the lubrication of hypodermic needles. Even over-the-counter indigestion remedies contain silicone that is absorbed by the stomach. No documented health hazards have ever been proven to result from the presence of small quantities of silicone in the body.

Rupture of the implant Rupture is extremely rare with modern implants. The actual incidence is unknown and research is ongoing. Rupture can result from deterioration of the implant shell over time, undetected damage at operation, a manufacturing flaw or a severe trauma to the chest.

If there is an internal or intracapsular rupture, there may be no dramatic change in the breast as the gel is still contained in the fibrous capsule.

If there is spread of the gel through the ruptured shell beyond the fibrous capsule (extracapsular spread), the rupture will be more obvious, with a change in the shape of the implant and possibly a reduction in the size due to extrusion of gel beyond the breast area. In the vast majority of extracapsular ruptures, the gel is still in the region of the original pocket and can be removed with the ruptured implant.

In a small number of cases, gel has been found in breast tissue itself, chest muscles, armpits, armpit glands, and around the nerves of the armpit. Removal may be necessary from these sites. Gel outside the capsule can cause inflammation with the development of lumps that can be felt.

However you should be reassured that normal activity will not cause a rupture. You can lie and sleep on your front and need not take any special precautions to ensure the integrity of your implants.

It is possible for implant rupture and leakage to occur undetected, as more often than not there are no symptoms or visible effects. Modern ultrasound machines are extremely accurate in determining if an implant is ruptured or is leaking, but are not 100 per cent reliable. MRI scans are reputedly more accurate, but few people in our experience undergo this investigation to determine implant integrity.

If you suffer a severe trauma to the chest e.g. following a car crash, you should undergo investigation until there is conclusive proof that your implants are intact. The ultimate proof of implant integrity is at operation when the implant can be removed for examination. It can be an extremely difficult decision to make to re-operate on suspicion of a ruptured or leaking implant as there is nothing more frustrating for you and your surgeon if the result at surgery shows no damage.

Rejection True rejection of the implant is extremely rare. However, if the wound becomes infected and breaks down, the implant will protrude from its pocket and will need to be removed until the infection has subsided before it can be re-inserted again. This is not true rejection, but a result of infection.

Implant lifespan It must be emphasised that breast implants are not guaranteed for life. There is ongoing debate and research regarding how long implants should be left in the body before being changed.

In the main, all patients should be investigated after a time to determine the integrity of their implants. Most surgeons would agree that a scan after 10 years, if not before, is a wise precaution. Most schools of thought would advocate a change of implants after 15 years. Research is ongoing. Generally, if you are still happy with your implants after many years, and they are not giving any symptoms, there is little reason to change them.

The risk of cancer Unfortunately, cancer of the breast is a common disease. Statistically, one in 12 women in the UK will develop breast cancer. Extensive worldwide research has conclusively demonstrated that there is no evidence that silicone breast implants increase the chance of future development of breast cancer; indeed, there is evidence that cancers don't grow as fast in patients with implants. Cancers also present earlier (because this group of patients is more breast aware, and breast lumps are easier to feel in the presence of an implant), so the survival rate of patients with implants who get breast cancer is better than those without.

We do however recommend that women who have a strong family history of breast cancer are vigilant in self-breast examination following surgery.

Flying and diving It is perfectly safe to fly in aircraft and go deep-sea diving without the risk of rupture of breast implants. Sudden extreme changes of pressure can cause implant rupture.

Removal of implant Before undergoing breast augmentation, many women express concern about the possibility of the effects of implant removal at some point in the future. Although breast augmentation is one of the very few operations in the surgical textbook that is readily reversible, very few of our patients have subsequently requested removal of their implants.

The commonest reason for implant removal is severe capsular contracture (see above) causing symptoms (pain and discomfort) and an undesirable shape and consistency.

The resulting size, shape and appearance of the breasts will very much depend on the preoperative state as well as age, skin tone and the amount of remaining breast tissue. It must be remembered that the actual breast tissue will shrink in size with increasing age, weight loss, hormonal changes etc. The implant will remain the same size.

Women who had a lot of loose skin before surgery have an increased chance of being left with thin, ptotic (droopy) breasts. It usually takes several weeks before the breasts will settle to their final shape following implant removal.

Postoperative management

Many surgeons recommend that a properly fitted bra be worn day and night for two weeks after surgery. Thereafter a bra should be worn as usual. Breasts that were droopy before the operation will droop more after the insertion of implants because of the increase in weight of the breasts. A properly fitted support bra should help prevent the breasts from drooping.

Some women find that wearing a bra in the postoperative period eases discomfort and some think it adds to it. Some surgeons are of the opinion that wearing bras in the immediate postoperative period increases the risk of future capsular contracture (see above).

The wound dressing should be kept dry and patients should wash themselves with a sponge, avoiding baths and showers until the incisions have properly healed.

Some surgeons advocate daily breast massage after the operation to reduce the chance of capsular contracture.

Heavy lifting should be avoided for two weeks after surgery. Strenuous exercise such as aerobics and swimming should be avoided for at least six weeks in order to give the wounds adequate time to heal fully.

Sutures are usually removed after seven to 10 days.

Recovery time Most women undergoing this operation are young and fit and tend to recover very quickly. Unless their occupation entails strenuous activity or heavy lifting, most women can go back to work after a few days. Office work can usually be resumed within a few days.

Results

Breast augmentation boosts the self-confidence of women who have previously felt inadequate in certain clothes, on the beach or in sexual relationships. Research has shown that there is a significant psychological benefit; over 90 per cent of women have increased self esteem and feeling of self worth following the operation, due to a more balanced perception of their body image. Most women are completely comfortable with the change to their breasts and cease to be aware of the implants after a few weeks.

With modern technology the newer breast implants now available have markedly reduced the incidence of capsule contracture (see above), which is the one major problem that could mar an otherwise perfect result.

The safety of silicone breast implants

In 1997, at the request of Her Majesty's Government, the Independent Review Group (IRG) was established to investigate the possible health risks associated with silicone breast implants and to examine the issues relating to preoperative patient information. The IRG published its findings in July 1998 and these are their conclusions:

1. There is no medical evidence for an abnormal immune response to silicone from breast implants in tissue.

2. There is no evidence for any link between silicone breast implants and any established connective tissue or autoimmune disease. If there is a risk, it is too small to be quantified.

3. Good evidence for the existence of a typical connective tissue or autoimmune disease or undefined conditions, such as 'silicone poisoning', is lacking. It is possible that other conditions such as low-grade chronic infection may account for some of the non-specific illnesses noted in some women with silicone gel implants.

4. The overall biological response to silicone is consistent with conventional forms of response to foreign materials, rather than an unusual toxic reaction.

5. There is no evidence that children of women with breast implants are at an increased risk of connective tissue disease.

6. The IRG recognised that there were issues such as the precise incidence of rupture where the scientific data was incomplete so that rigorous conclusions could not be drawn.

Despite all the scientific evidence currently available, which clearly demonstrates that silicone implants do no harm to the body, there are those who still question the facts.

The question 'Are silicone breast implants safe?' cannot be answered with a simple yes/no reply. 'Safety' is not a simple, absolute concept. It is widely accepted to mean 'freedom from an undue risk of harm'. The word 'undue' is critical. It is impossible to guarantee that any given set of conditions can be completely free from any possibility of harm. This is particularly pertinent to medical practice, where all deliberate invasive procedures carry some risk to health.

If silicone implants were indeed dangerous to health then all surgeons who perform this procedure to any extent would be seeing large numbers of patients with symptoms or established diseases. In reality this is not the case.

In summary it can be stated that with long-term experience and current knowledge available, patients who contemplate having breast enlargement should not be apprehensive. The likelihood of developing any serious illness or condition following implantation of silicone implants is extremely remote.

Breast Uplift

A breast uplift or mastopexy operation will reshape a sagging (ptotic) breast to a more normal, pleasing and youthful shape without changing its actual size. A new 'skin bra' is fashioned which reduces the surface area of the skin covering the breasts in relation to the breast volume so that they are fuller and not so saggy. The nipples are lifted to a higher position and this gives the breast a more pleasing, youthful shape.

There are varying degrees of sagging (ptosis) of breasts. The degree of ptosis is measured according to the position and level of the nipple to the level of the crease under the breast.

The most common reason for having the operation is actual loss of breast substance (volume) following pregnancy or weight loss. The amount of skin covering the breast remains the same. With less breast substance to cover, the breasts become droopy with the nipples lying lower than the breast crease on standing. If the nipple is above the crease then breast augmentation is a better operation.

The reason the breasts tend to droop after pregnancy is because the glandular tissue increases in size under the effect of hormones and displaces the fatty tissue. At the same time the support of the breasts softens as part of the general stretching of fibrous tissue in the body. After breast-feeding, or even if it is not started, the gland tissue goes back to its normal size, but the fat tissue isn't replaced. The net result is a softer, lower breast.

Sometimes there may not be an actual reduction of breast size. Repeated pregnancies will stretch breast skin resulting in loss of tone of the skin covering the breasts. The loss of tone of the covering breast skin will give a more droopy appearance.

If the breasts are droopy simply because they are very bulky then a breast reduction should be performed. This combines the skin tightening and nipple raising operation with removal of breast tissue. If, on the other hand, the breasts are still going to be too small even if they are raised to a better position, then mastopexy can be combined with augmentation.

There are no exercises that are capable of shrinking stretched skin. A good supporting bra, worn routinely (especially during pregnancy) is the best form of prevention. During late pregnancy it is a good idea to wear a support bra day and night, and to wear increasing bra sizes as the breasts increase, so that they always fit well. After pregnancy the same series of bras can be worn in reverse order. The idea is to keep the breasts well supported at all times. This reduces the stretching of the breast support fibres.

The preoperative consultation

It is perhaps worth emphasising that this is not an operation that is favoured by every woman who is concerned with her droopy breasts; many decline this procedure once they realise the extent of the scarring. It is not to everyone's liking and the first postoperative year especially can lead to problems in a patient's relationship, which is why we try to ensure that wherever possible or appropriate the patient's partner is always present at the consultation.

Extensive scarring as a result of a breast uplift will always be visible no matter how well the skin heals, even though the scars will usually fade in the fullness of time. Scars can stretch on occasions and be very noticeable, so it is important that you fully take this into consideration. We usually show serial photographs of the appearance at intervals following surgery. You may wish to go away and think again before returning for another consultation. You may decide that the current appearance of your breasts is preferable to the likely postoperative appearance and scarring. Or you may decide that the scarring is an acceptable trade-off for better breast shape.

This surgery is not suitable for everyone. For example, pregnancy must be avoided for some years after the operation to avoid stretching the scars, so this operation should really only be considered after your family is complete.

You are advised to make a list of questons to ask the surgeon in the unlikely event that he does not cover the important issues. You should ask about the following:

1. The extent of scarring and the technique he will use. In addition the likely size and shape afterwards.
2. Postoperative care and the recovery period.
3. The psychological effects the extensive scarring on the front of and underneath the breasts has generally had on previous patients.
4. What happens if you get pregnant afterwards.

5. Breast-feeding.

6. Pre- and post-operative photographs. Ask to be shown examples of previous work at intervals after the operation.

The operation

Before the operation, great care is taken to mark out the precise areas of skin excision, which will effectively enable your surgeon to construct a new 'skin bra' and raise the nipple to an elevated position. No breast tissue is removed.

You will be admitted on the morning of the surgery. The operation is usually performed under general anaesthetic (see pages 61–63). Several techniques are available and the one used will depend on the surgeon's preference as well as on the particular problem in question. Permanent scarring will always result.

Usually there is a scar around the circumference of the areola which continues from the lower edge of the areola in a vertical line down to join another curved scar (the length of which will vary from patient to patient) in the crease underneath the breast. After the wound is sutured, a padded dressing is applied and you will usually be discharged home the following day.

If there is only a small degree of droop it is possible to modify the technique and perform the operation so that the final scar is situated at the circumference of the areola only, thereby eliminating all the scarring below the areola in the lower half of the breast.

After the operation a support dressing is applied, which is left on for several days.

Postoperative events

Scars This is the main problem with this operation. Although your surgeon will try to make the wound look as neat as possible, it is unlikely that the scar will ever completely disappear. They may even stretch or become red and raised and require further treatment in the future (see 'Improving Unsightly Scars', pages 196–199).

The unfavourable appearance of the scars can take up to two years and possibly longer to settle before they fade so you will need to be patient about this. This should all be discussed with you at your preoperative consultation.

Infection and postoperative bleeding This is a possibility, as it is after any surgical procedure.

Soreness and pain This is likely to be present after the operation but it is not usually severe. It can usually be managed with oral painkillers.

Immediate results At the time the dressings are first removed and you see the results for the first time the shape of the breasts is often quite peculiar, with the lower part of the breast, below the nipple, having a rather flattened appearance. This settles into a more natural shape in a few months due to moulding by the wearing of a bra and gravity.

Recurrence In some patients there is a risk that the breasts will become droopy again. Wearing a well-fitting support bra reduces the likelihood of this happening. Recurrence of droopiness generally occurs following further pregnancies, weight gain and failure to adequately support large breasts postoperatively.

Sensory changes Sensitivity of the nipples may be reduced or altered although in all but a tiny minority of women this will return to normal.

Breast-feeding After a mastopexy operation there should be no trouble with breast-feeding. Pregnancy itself, however, must be avoided for some years after the operation to avoid stretching the scars. This operation is thus best carried out only after your family is complete.

Postoperative management

You are strongly advised to wear a properly fitted support bra night and day for some weeks. This supports the skin, helps the healing process and gently moulds the shape of the breasts during recovery.

The dressings must be kept clean, dry and intact until they are removed about a week after the surgery. Strenuous movements should be avoided for several weeks and driving is discouraged for two weeks, to avoid shear stress on the wounds, which can be fragile. After the dressings have been removed the scars can be massaged with skin cream.

Results

In carefully selected patients, and with optimum healing of the scars, the results of mastopexy are very pleasing. As long as the breasts are not too large and are supported most of the time, most women find they can wear strappy tops with confidence, something they may not have been able to do for years.

You should think very carefully before undergoing this procedure and discuss it with your partner, as the final scarring may be unacceptable to some. This is an operation with a prolonged recovery period. It takes many months for the final result to be seen and is not recommended for a young woman who is likely to have more children.

If you get pregnant following this operation, be prepared for the scars to stretch and accept that the breasts may well become droopy again. Although a further uplift can be performed, you may well regret having the original surgery before completing your family.

BREAST REDUCTION

Large breasts can be a source of major embarrassment and discomfort. As well as the difficulty of finding clothes that fit and look elegant, they tend to interfere with active sports. Sometimes they also cause backache and their weight makes bra straps dig in over the shoulders. They can cause skin problems in the crease below each breast. With the passage of time they will hang lower and lower and the skin can become covered in stretch marks.

If very large breasts are simply an expression of generalised obesity then simple loss of weight, or obesity surgery might be a better treatment, at least in the first instance.

Most women who have any sort of cosmetic surgery simply wish to approach a 'norm' of appearance. For example, those with an unusually prominent nose wish to reduce its size somewhat; those with tiny breasts simply wish to increase them to a size proportionate to the rest of their body. This motivation is especially relevant in the case of women with very large breasts. The aim of the operation is to make the breasts a B or C bra-cup size, whatever size they were before.

The preoperative consultation

The surgeon will discuss all relevant and important issues pertaining to this operation with you at a preoperative consultation. In the unlikely event that he omits certain points or issues, be prepared to ask about the following:

1. Technique used
2. Extent of scarring
3. Duration of operation
4. Recovery time

5. Likelihood of complications, e.g. nipple loss (necrosis), sensory loss to nipples, infection.
6. Breast-feeding afterwards.

The operation

Breast reduction is performed along similar lines to mastopexy (see above), with the addition of the precise removal of breast tissue. Thus a new skin bra is created that leaves the nipple at an elevated position as well as creating smaller, more youthful looking breasts.

Reducing the size of the breasts is a major operation. Several different techniques are used but they all cause quite significant scarring. The most usual method leaves a scar that runs around the edge of the areola and one in the crease underneath the breast with a vertical scar linking the two. These scars do not usually show outside an ordinary bra or bikini top. Although in most patients they fade with time, they should be considered to be permanent.

You will generally be admitted on the morning of the operation. Because this is major surgery, preoperative health checks have to be very thorough. Photographs will be taken and the new site for the nipples marked. The usual position of the nipple is about 22cm (8 1/2in) along the breast axis. The breast axis is a line that starts one third of the way along the collarbone, from its origin at the upper end of the breast bone (sternum) and descends downwards and outwards to bisect the main bulk of the breast. The nipple is usually on this line or just lateral to it (on the outer side of it).

A breast reduction is a mastopexy (see above, pages 157–161) combined with the removal of an accurately measured wedge of breast tissue. The volume of breast tissue removed is predetermined by accurately marking out the breasts beforehand when you are standing up. The preoperative markings used in breast reduction are specifically designed to reduce a three dimensional structure in an accurate and symmetrical manner.

Several different techniques for breast reduction have been developed. The specific technique used will depend on the particular situation, the surgeon's preference as well your consent and preference.

All breast-reduction techniques are designed to preserve the 'viability' of the nipple. This means that in repositioning the nipple to its new elevated site, the blood supply must be preserved. This is usually achieved by ensuring that the nipple-areola complex is attached to an adequate bridge of skin, which will provide it with a sufficient blood supply to ensure its survival.

In very large breasts, the nipple-areola complex can be removed completely and resutured to its new site as a free skin graft. In expert hands this technique works very well, and the graft usually takes successfully. If not, either the entire graft or part of it will die, often requiring further surgery at a later time (see below).

Most sutures are placed under the skin and are dissolvable. All other sutures on the skin surface are removed after about seven to 10 days.

Postoperative events

Partial or total loss of nipple This occurs if, following the operation, the blood supply to the nipple-areola complex is inadequate. The nipple-areola complex may turn dark or black in colour, usually very soon after surgery, and gradually shrink in size over the next few days or weeks, or it may ulcerate at some stage until it eventually heals to a smaller size. If this happens, it will need to be reconstructed if the patient requests so. Problems with the blood supply to the nipples are more common in cases where a massive reduction has been done, or if the patient smokes. Being too active after the operation or otherwise not adhering to the postoperative instructions can also endanger the viability of the nipples.

Swelling and bruising The breasts will be swollen and probably quite bruised and tender for a few days after surgery, and will need to be supported well by wearing a supportive and well-fitting bra.

Soreness and pain Pain and discomfort are likely in the immediate postoperative phase but are not usually severe. Standard painkillers control any discomfort or pain postoperatively.

Bleeding and infection This is a possibility, as it is after any surgical procedure.

Scars Scars may stretch and become red and raised. If the scars do not heal well they can generally be improved about a year after the original operation (see 'Improving Unsightly Scars', pages 196–199). Every attempt is made to make the scars as neat and inconspicuous as possible, but they will always show on close examination.

Sensory changes Sensitivity of the nipples is usually reduced. Most patients with very large breasts do not have much sensation in the nipples preoperatively. Sometimes a range of strange sensations, such as pins and needles, burning or stabbing pains are experienced. These last for a few months and slowly return to normal.

Breast shape   The breasts may look quite odd initially, with a flattened shape beneath the nipple, which may look too low; as time passes they will settle down to look more natural. It is unlikely that the breasts will have a perfect shape or be exactly symmetrical.

Inverted nipples   Sometimes one or both nipples can become inverted after the operation. Further surgery can be performed to correct this if the patient wishes (see below, pages 165–167).

Recurrence   There have been cases where further enlargement has occurred after surgery, but as long as there is not excessive weight gain this is a very unlikely event.

Breast-feeding   It is unlikely that a baby could be successfully breast-fed afterwards. Indeed, it is very important that pregnancy itself is avoided for several years because the scars will stretch badly during pregnancy unless they are completely mature.

Postoperative management
You are strongly advised to wear a properly fitted support bra night and day for some weeks. This supports the skin and helps the healing and gently moulds the shape of the breasts during recovery.

The dressings must be kept clean, dry and intact until they are removed. Strenuous movements should be avoided for several weeks and driving is discouraged for two weeks. After the dressings are removed the scars can be massaged with skin cream.

Results
The initial result after breast reduction is often a very peculiar shape, with a reduced distance between the nipple and both the fold under the breast and the main bulk of the breast above the nipple. Gradually, over the next few months, gravity and the moulding effect of the wearing of a bra produce the final shape. It can often take up to a year before the final result is seen. Adjustments to the scar (see 'Improving Unsightly Scars', pages 196–199) or touch-up operations to improve the shape can be done if necessary after this time.

As with a breast uplift procedure, all patients must appreciate and be prepared for the consequences of a further pregnancy afterwards. The scars may well stretch, especially if there is a large increase in breast size during pregnancy and further ptosis (droop) may well occur. Some women may be able to breast-feed afterwards, although be prepared for the fact that this is not possible in most cases.

Some surgeons have described this operation as one of the most gratifying of all cosmetic surgeries, with an extremely high success rate despite the extensive scarring. Patients say that it is like an enormous weight (literally!) has been lifted. You can go on the beach without embarrassment and fit into ordinary clothes. After the operation most women feel a tremendous sense of freedom because they can do all the things that their large breasts prevented them doing before.

THE CORRECTION OF INVERTED NIPPLES

Nipple inversion is an embarrassing condition affecting about two per cent of all women. In the majority of cases, inverted nipples occur as a result of a congenital defect caused by an underdevelopment of the milk ducts, which retract the nipples as the breast develops. This condition can also be acquired after certain breast diseases e.g. mastitis, breast cancer or following breast surgery (see above, page 164).

The classification of nipple inversion
Nipple inversion is classified into three grades according to the severity of the condition.

- Grade 1: can be pulled out easily and maintain this projection. This type will also respond to external stimulation.
- Grade 2: can be relatively easily pulled out but have a tendency to retract easily.
- Grade 3: is severely retracted and difficult to pull out manually.

Little suction devices that attach to the nipples are available, which can be used to treat inverted nipples. They are only likely to be successful if the nipples come out easily (Grade 1). Some women have found that Grade 1 inversion corrects after childbirth.

The preoperative consultation

Make sure the surgeon covers the following points:

1. Technique used.
2. The incidence of recurrence.
3. Sensory loss to nipples.
4. Breast-feeding.
5. The cost of further revision surgery.

The operation

Many techniques have been developed to correct this deformity. There is currently no consensus of opinion as to which method is the best, as none exists which is 100 per cent successful. All techniques are performed through incisions at the base of the nipple or in the areola margin.

Surgery to correct inverted nipples can usually be performed under local anaesthetic on a day-care basis. Occasionally an overnight stay in a clinic may be recommended.

The technique used will depend on the severity of the inversion and the surgeon's preference after a detailed discussion with you.

One of the commonest techniques used involves making a narrow incision at the base of the nipple and cutting through the fibres and milk ducts, which pull the nipple inwards. This releases (everts) the nipple outwards. Further tiny stab incisions are made at the base of the nipple. Stitches are then inserted via these stab incisions, which when pulled tight will close the tissue defect beneath the nipple in an attempt to prevent it from inverting. Other techniques for correcting inverted nipples use longer incisions, either at the base of the nipple or along the outer margin of the areola. All techniques attempt to release the constricting bands of tissue, which pull the nipple inwards and close the hollow space beneath the nipple to prevent it from inverting.

Some surgeons inject filler material in the nipple, to make it larger if necessary, either at the time of the operation or afterwards in a second separate procedure.

Postoperative management

Breast-feeding Breast-feeding may prove difficult if not impossible after this surgery, due to the fact that the milk ducts in the nipple are often irreparably damaged by the operation. However the breast ducts do have very good powers of regeneration, so although breast-feeding is not necessarily entirely ruled out by this surgery, it should still be regarded as such by all who undergo this procedure in order to avoid disappointment. Obviously this will be a prime factor in your decision to have surgery in the first place.

Sensory changes Sensation in the nipple may be partially or even totally impaired. This may be permanent, but is very rare. Most women usually experience some loss of sensation, which gradually returns to normal.

Recurrence or failure It is still possible for the nipples to invert again after the operation, even after the most expert surgery. A further correction may be required. Recurrence is a problem usually in those cases that were severely inverted, i.e. Grade 3 preoperatively. Correction of Grades 1 and 2 is generally very successful.

In some cases, recurrence of nipple inversion can still occur several years after what was originally deemed a successful operation. Most recurrences, however, occur within a few weeks of the original procedure.

Results

The usual result is entirely normal-looking nipples which react normally to temperature changes and being touched. Scarring is minimal and usually does not present a problem.

Body-Contour Surgery

LIPOSUCTION

Liposuction (fat suction) was popularised in the early 1980s and has completely revolutionised body-contour surgery. It was initially developed to resculpture parts of the body that had unsightly stubborn areas of fat, which did not respond to diet or exercise. Up until that time the only technique available entailed a wedge excision of an area of fat, which resulted in unfavourable scars. It was our opinion at that time that the aesthetic result was no better than the previous situation and in many ways could be deemed worse.

Various factions of interested parties have attempted to rename or modify the liposuction procedure leading to much confusion in nomenclature. Terms such as 'spot fat reduction', 'liposculpture', 'fat contouring' and 'lipoplasty' add to the confusion. Essentially the procedure entails the removal of localised areas of body fat by sucking it out. For the purpose of this chapter we refer to this procedure as liposuction, although the other terms named above mean exactly the same thing.

When this procedure was first popularised by Dr Gerard Illouz in Paris in the early 1980s a maximum limit of two litres of pure fat was recommended to be removed at any one treatment session. This was to ensure maximum safety for the patient as excessive fat removal could lead to excessive postoperative bleeding together with its associated dangers.

In recent years, however, some surgeons have started treating patients who are seriously overweight. These surgeons boast of routinely removing up to 15 litres or more of fat in one operation. This technique is popularly known as 'megaliposculpture' or 'high-volume lipoplasty'. It is still controversial with regard to its overall safety, as most surgeons will not remove such large quantities of fat in one procedure.

Liposuction can benefit many patients where previous techniques of body contouring have proved inadequate in achieving the desired result. It can also be combined with other standard procedures, thereby producing better and longer lasting results: for example, it can be used as part of a facelift procedure or abdominoplasty.

Liposuction is most effective in those patients who are of normal weight, but who have stubborn areas of fat. It is not a substitute for weight loss in the obese.

This technique is used to reshape or resculpture the following areas of the body:

- Face and neck: In particular, the double chin and fatty neck. It is routinely used in conjunction with a facelift procedure in patients with excess fat under the chin and in the neck.
- Limbs: Thighs (riding breeches deformity), knees, calves, ankles, buttocks, fat arms and other abnormal isolated fat deposits.
- Abdomen: Used alone in suitable cases or in conjunction with a tummy tuck.
- Breasts: Abnormal collections of fat in breasts.
- Lipomas: Large isolated collections of fat.

Available Techniques

Traditional technique

This method involves using a blunt metal cannula (surgical tube) to suck out the offending fat using a high negative-pressure pump. Over the years variations in technique have appeared. One of the most popular and successful of these has been the use of specially designed syringes to suck out the offending fat thereby eliminating the use of electric suction pumps.

Ultrasonic technique

This technique utilises high-frequency ultrasonic energy emitted from a surgical probe. The ultrasonic energy is emitted at a pre-set frequency, which ruptures or dissolves the fat cells, releasing the fat stored inside the cells before it is gently sucked out.

The frequency required to rupture the fat cells is not sufficient to cause damage to surrounding tissues such as muscles, bones, tendons and blood vessels.

This technique is widely regarded as being gentler than the traditional method described above, and many authorities will argue that there is less discomfort, bruising and swelling afterwards. In addition, it is claimed that this method achieves a smoother skin surface, tightens loose skin and eliminates or at least greatly improves the 'orange-peel' effect of cellulite.

Laser-assisted liposuction

This is a technique that may gain approval in the UK in the near future as it is currently gaining popularity in the USA.

Prior to suction, a cold laser is passed over the area to be treated for several minutes. The laser liquefies the fat and facilitates easier removal. There is little or no risk of damage to the skin and surrounding tissues, as this is a cold laser. This procedure takes less time than the traditional method.

There is less postoperative bruising and swelling, less pain and discomfort and therefore a shorter recovery time. Although results are still being evaluated, more experienced surgeons are claiming better results than those achieved with the traditional technique alone. Only time will tell.

Nature of operation

You will be admitted on the morning of the operation. Large areas are best treated using general anaesthesia. Small areas can be treated using local anaesthesia and sedation. The areas to be treated are carefully marked with marker pen on the skin, with the patient's agreement, and photographs are taken.

Small stab incisions of a few millimetres are made at strategic points on the skin surface for the insertion of the cannula (or surgical probe if using the ultrasonic technique).

The area to be operated on is first infiltrated with saline solution containing local anaesthetic and a vasoconstrictor (blood-vessel constricting) agent, usually adrenaline. A large volume of fluid is injected and this is commonly known as the 'tumescent' technique. The purpose of this injection is to facilitate fat removal, reduce intra and postoperative bleeding and postoperative pain and discomfort. Some surgeons don't inject any fluid – this is called the 'dry' technique. There is little difference in the results obtained, although after the dry technique much less fluid seeps out of the incisions.

Fat is generally removed in layers in tunnels using appropriate cannulae. There are many different cannulae available nowadays and each surgeon will select the one that best suits the situation.

Once all the fat is removed the incisions are sutured and usually a specially designed pressure garment is fitted. The length of stay in clinic is usually no longer than one night.

Postoperative events

Bruising and swelling These are inevitable in the immediate postoperative period and it is not unusual for the operated area to look larger as a result. Most of the bruising and swelling will subside within seven to 10 days, but in a few patients it can last for months.

Scars Scars are generally small and wherever possible are placed at inconspicuous sites. Whereas a permanent mark will always remain, it should not cause you any long-term concern.

Rippling, looseness and sagging of the skin This can occur if either excessive amounts of fat have to be removed from an area, or if the skin is of such a poor tone initially that removing even a small amount of fat will exacerbate this effect. Although each case must be assessed on its own merits, as a general guide, those patients who are under the age of 35 years old have a much better chance of a satisfactory result.

It is impossible to predict accurately how much the skin will tighten up after the operation. Some women will not accept loose skin in return for a more pleasing contour whereas others will do so quite happily, so this is something you must consider carefully before treatment. Skin does not contain any voluntary muscle so no amount of exercising will increase its tone or tighten it.

At present surgery is the only effective way of tightening loose skin once it has stretched sufficiently to lose its elasticity. The final resting state of the skin is variable, and dependent on the unique physiology of the individual.

Lumpiness and hardness This usually occurs for a while after the operation and is part of the normal healing process. The fat is removed in layers in tunnels. These tunnels fill up with blood, which subsequently clots, causing hardness. The speed with which the body dissolves and then absorbs the clotted blood will determine how long the hardness lasts.

In addition, during the healing process a certain amount of scar tissue will be formed in the fatty tissue where the tunnels were made under the skin. This will add to the overall bulk of the remaining fatty tissue. This scar tissue will soften and reduce in volume with time so it will take several months before the final result is achieved. Rarely, an excessive amount of scar tissue will be formed causing an extended period of hardness and discomfort.

Ruts, depressions and defects These can occur as a result of too much fat having been removed from a particular area or site. Although this complication can occur with any surgeon it is much less common in experienced hands. A further procedure may be required to improve the situation.

Correcting ruts and defects will entail filling in defects with fat taken from a suitable donor site in the body. Sometimes several procedures are required as some of the transferred fat will dissolve and be absorbed.

Asymmetry It is not possible to promise perfect symmetry after the operation, as the body is asymmetrical to begin with. Where an obvious asymmetry results, further surgery may be necessary to correct it.

Skin loss Rarely, small patches of skin may die, especially near incision sites, resulting in scar formation. Scar revision (see 'Improving Unsightly Scars', pages 196–199) will usually improve the situation.

Numbness Changes in sensation can occur in the treated area due to nerve damage and may take some time to resolve completely. Various sensations have been described by patients such as stiffness, pins and needles, electric-shock-like sensations and persistent discomfort. These undesirable symptoms generally settle in time.

Blood transfusion This is rarely required. A blood transfusion is only necessary if too much bleeding has occurred into the surrounding tissues, usually as a result of trying to remove too much fat.

Postoperative management

Over the years there have been several reported cases in the press of patients collapsing at home following liposuction, with the occasional fatality. These cases have usually referred to those patients who have been discharged from hospital or clinic too soon or who have not received adequate postoperative care. Such complications can be avoided with proper postoperative care.

All patients who have had large volumes of fat removed should be carefully monitored for at least 24 hours after their operation. You should receive adequate pain relief and fluid replacement. In this way serious postoperative complications can usually be avoided.

You will be advised to rest for the first 24 to 48 hours after discharge from hospital. There is usually a degree of stiffness and discomfort. After this time you are encouraged to become more active.

Most surgeons usually recommend an elastic garment, which should be worn for several weeks. The purpose of the support garment is to reduce bruising and swelling in the immediate postoperative period, and to support the re-sculptured tissues in the ensuing weeks in order to maintain their final favourable shape. There is a wide variety of liposuction garments now available for all areas of the body.

Showers and baths can be taken as early as the second day after surgery. Apart from when washing, the support garment should be worn at all times in the first 10 days. After that, it should be worn during the day for the next three weeks.

Failure to wear a correctly fitted support garment can result in contour defects which may be difficult to correct afterwards.

Gentle massage of the treated areas should begin about 10 days after the operation. Some surgeons advocate ultrasound or other physiotherapy to disperse the bruising and swelling (which can be quite pronounced) more quickly. Sutures are usually removed after a week.

Results
Once removed, the fat should not return. This is because the fat cells have been permanently removed from the area. The remaining fat cells in that area will not have the capacity to absorb sufficient fat in future to return to the previous large volume.

If your calorific intake is excessive after the procedure, fat will continue to be deposited in the body, but only in those areas that were not operated on. You should still watch your weight carefully after the operation. If a lot of weight is gained the treated areas are prone to become lumpy and uneven.

Liposuction is an extremely successful operation that permanently removes unwanted pads of unsightly fat.

It is difficult at present to predict how the newer ultrasonic liposuction techniques will be accepted by surgeons and patients. We have tried these techniques and find the traditional technique superior; results in our hands are very successful.

TUMMY TUCK, ABDOMINAL REDUCTION
(ABDOMINOPLASTY, ABDOMINAL LIPECTOMY)

The tummy tuck operation is designed to tighten the loose skin and muscles of the abdomen following pregnancy and weight loss. It should leave as short a transverse scar as possible in the lower abdomen below the bikini line. It is not an operation to treat obesity. There will usually be only a small amount of weight loss but a significantly improved shape.

Various techniques have been described over the years, but the primary difference in the popular techniques widely practised today is the shape and length of the skin incision.

Many surgeons carry out liposuction in conjunction with the standard 'tummy tuck' procedure in suitable cases, as the final result is superior. We do not recommend extensive liposuction in an overweight person at the same time as the abdominoplasty procedure as there is a serious risk of damaging the blood supply to the abdominal flap leading to tissue necrosis (loss). In such situations it is perhaps best to perform the procedure in two stages.

Patients who have lost massive amounts of weight often have an apron of skin hanging down in front of the abdomen. They often find that they get skin problems such as chafing and rashes under this apron, which are difficult to control.

Apart from improving the profile, the procedure also helps to remove stretch marks and scars from the lower part of the abdomen. It must be stressed that in some skin types, stretching the skin as part of the operative procedure can produce fresh stretch marks even above the navel.

Abdominal muscle exercises will help to tone up the muscles following pregnancy but will not tighten loose skin or the postpartum 'pot belly', which is caused by muscular diastasis (see below).

Choosing the correct procedure

The procedure selected for a particular patient will depend on the circumstances; each has advantages and disadvantages. All the options should be explained to you, and your preference will also be taken into consideration.

A long, horizontal, lower-abdominal incision that gives a scar whose mid point lies just at the upper border of the 'pubic bone' is the incision of choice with most surgeons. In this situation the raised abdominal flap should be lax enough to stretch downwards so that the skin at the upper extremity of the umbilicus (belly button) can be pulled down far enough to reach the suprapubic skin incision. If this cannot be achieved without undue tension on the abdominal flap a lower vertical midline scar will result as well. There is quite often a deep crease underneath the overhanging flap and most surgeons place the scar in this crease.

Where there is horizontal tissue laxity as well, a vertical midline incision with accompanying scar will be necessary in addition to the horizontal scar.

This operation is not suitable if you are planning future pregnancies, or if you have previous unfavourable scarring that may compromise the viability of the abdominal flap.

Preoperative evaluation
Most women who seek this procedure do so for one or several of the following reasons:

1. Being embarrassed wearing swimwear because of visible bulges.
   Visible stretch marks, sagging skin and wrinkles if wearing a bikini.
2. Difficulty getting clothing, which hides or diminishes a protrusion or bulges.
3. Limitation of social, leisure and sexual activities to avoid embarrassment.

When examining your abdomen, the surgeon will assess the amount of loose skin, stretch marks, the distribution of fat in the abdominal wall and flanks and whether there is an apron of fat and skin present. In addition the degree of muscle laxity following any previous pregnancies is important to note. It may be that the vertical midline (rectus abdominis) muscles have separated (muscular diastasis) and need meticulous repair to bring them back together as normal.

With you lying flat on your back the degree of soft-tissue (fat and skin) laxity is determined by attempting to oppose, by a pinching manoeuvre with both hands, the skin at the upper level of the umbilicus to the upper limit of the pubic bone. If this is easily achieved, then an additional vertical scar will probably be unnecessary. If this is not the case, then a vertical scar will almost certainly be necessary if a low transverse incision is used. Your surgeon should explain this carefully to you in order to avoid any postoperative disappointment.

With you standing up, the degree of abdominal protrusion, laxity, wrinkling, and excess hanging skin and fat (apron) is noted and recorded. It is usually on standing that these deformities are most prominent, as they tend to be less obvious on lying down.

The presence of abdominal scars following any previous surgery is noted and evaluated. Horizontal scars in the upper abdomen, which will not be removed at operation, or in the lower abdomen may present a potential hazard regarding a reduced tissue circulation to the lower extremity of the abdominal flap leading to flap necrosis (see above).

Preoperative photographs will be taken of front and back views as well as both side-profile views.

The operation

You will be admitted on the morning of surgery. A general anaesthetic is usually necessary although some surgeons operate using an epidural anaesthetic (see page 61) with sedation. In selected cases fat is sucked away from the abdomen first by liposuction (see above, pages 168–173). A long horizontal incision is made in the lower abdomen below the so-called bikini line. The skin-fat flap is dissected (lifted) from the muscles of the abdomen as far upwards as the rib cage and lower aspect of the breastbone.

An incision is then made around the whole circumference of the umbilicus (navel) and it is freed from its attachments to the skin and fat of the abdominal wall. It has the appearance of a 'mushroom on a stalk'.

The abdominal muscles are usually tightened with non-dissolvable stitches, as invariably they have been stretched. The excess skin and fat layer is stretched and re-draped downwards and the excess is suitably trimmed. Because the flap is stretched downwards, the wound is closed under tension so that the abdominal wall is as tight as possible. The umbilicus is re-sited, after a small circular area of skin at the new site of the umbilicus is removed, so that it effectively ends up in its original position. Dressings are applied to the incision lines.

Drains are usually inserted under the abdominal flap to suck out any blood and serum that collects in the space behind the flap in the first 24 to 48 hours following surgery. These are usually removed on the second postoperative day prior to discharge home.

While you are still asleep under anaesthetic, a heavy-duty elastic corset will be fitted to facilitate healing, enhance comfort and reduce the chances of a postoperative bleed.

Postoperative care

You will initially be nursed in bed with your knees and hips flexed, with pillows under your legs to ease tension on the abdominal wall and lessen discomfort.

Ankle- and knee-flexion exercises are encouraged and elastic stockings will be fitted to prevent postoperative deep vein thrombosis. Intermittently inflatable cuffs fitted around the calves and used in the first few hours following surgery are employed by many clinics to promote venous circulation, and further act to prevent venous thrombosis.

You will be encouraged to move about the following day with the aid of adequate pain relief. Initially oral fluids and a light diet are advised until you are able to tolerate solids fully, which is usually in the first few hours following surgery.

In selected cases some surgeons advocate inserting a catheter (rubber tube) into the bladder in the operating theatre just prior to surgery. This ensures that the bladder is empty throughout and facilitates wound closure at the conclusion of the operation. It also facilitates immediate postoperative nursing care, as patients do not need to endure the difficulties and discomfort of attempting to empty their bladder while still bedridden.

A bath or shower is permitted after five days. Gentle activities are resumed slowly in the first few days postoperatively. Vigorous activities such as sports, swimming, and going to the gym are permitted after six weeks.

Recovery time is very much dependent on the individual. Your return to work will also depend on the nature of surgery. As a general guideline, most women will achieve near normal activity after four to six weeks.

The length of stay in the clinic is usually no longer than two days and the sutures, if they are not dissolvable, are removed after about 10 days.

Postoperative events

Pain and discomfort This is usually most prominent in the first 48 hours after surgery. After that time most patients are fit to be looked after at home with appropriate medication. Because the tissues have been stitched under tension this procedure probably causes more pain and discomfort than any other cosmetic procedure.

Strong opiate analgesics are usually necessary in the immediate postoperative period in most patients. Thereafter oral painkillers or suppositories generally suffice.

Infection Wound infection can result in delayed healing. Sometimes complete wound breakdown (dehiscence) can occur requiring further surgery to resuture (stitch) the wound. As a result, an unfavourable scar may occur (see below) which may require revision (see 'Improving Unsightly Scars', pages 196–199) at a later date, usually after a few months.

Haematoma This is a collection of blood caused by bleeding occurring beneath the abdominal flap after the operation. It is a rare complication but, if severe, it will need to be evacuated (drained) under a general anaesthetic. A rapidly expanding haematoma can cause an increase in tension on the abdominal flap and compromise the circulation, thereby necessitating prompt action on the part of the surgeon.

Seroma This is a collection of fluid that has accumulated under the abdominal flap in the postoperative period. It can usually be removed easily with needle aspiration but this may need to be repeated several times as the accumulation of fluid can often recur before it finally resolves.

Stretch marks These will generally be removed if they lie below the umbilicus. In some skin types, stretching the abdominal flap after surgery can lead to new stretch-mark formation. These newly formed stretch marks may lie above the level of the umbilicus even if not present there previously. It is very important that your surgeon explains this, and that you take it on board, in order to avoid unnecessary disappointment afterwards.

Skin loss Thankfully, flap necrosis is extremely rare in abdominoplasty. It occurs as the result of an impaired circulation to the abdominal flap following surgery. This is particularly more likely to happen in heavy smokers (see page 48–49). It is more likely to occur if the flap has been closed under too much tension. It can also result from an expanding haematoma (see above) or even poor surgical technique.

Previous high transverse surgical scars or lower transverse scars, which have not been removed at surgery, will increase the risk of flap necrosis. By far the commonest cause of this complication nowadays is excessive liposuction to the abdominal flap prior to flap mobilisation.

Treatment for necrosis will depend on the extent and nature of the damage. The timing of further surgery is also important to appreciate. This varies from simple excision of dead tissue with closure of the defect wherever possible to wide excision with skin grafting. If treated conservatively with wound dressings even quite large defects gradually close on their own, which makes the revision operation much easier.

Scars Scars may become stretched or thickened (keloid) and may require revision (see 'Improving Unsightly Scars', pages 196–199) at a much later date if they do not settle in time. Steroid injections and silicone gel or sheets are used routinely in the first instance, with generally good results.

Loss of the navel This is a rare complication resulting from an inadequate blood supply to the navel after it has been re-sited to its new position in the abdominal flap. Further surgery may be required to reconstruct a new navel.

Malposition of the navel This rarely occurs and is most likely to be the result of surgical error. The new navel may be placed too high or low or not in the middle. Further surgery may be required to move it to a more favourable position.

Abdominal asymmetry This rare problem occurs if more tissue has been removed from one side than the other. Further surgery may be required to correct the difference.

Loss of sensation Most patients will experience a degree of sensory loss for several weeks to the lower half of the abdomen below the level of the navel. This results from the unavoidable damage to the sensory nerves that supply the area. These nerves regenerate slowly, and after several months sensation begins to return.

Results

A tummy tuck procedure will flatten and tone up a previously flabby stomach. All patients must be aware that a long horizontal scar will result, which may stretch or thicken and take time to mature fully. The results of the procedure can make a huge difference to self-esteem and confidence, and often encourage patients to adopt a healthier regime of diet and exercise.

Genital Cosmetic Surgery

Vaginal Tightening

After a vaginal delivery of a baby, many women feel that making love is not as pleasurable as it was before because the vagina has stretched. It is also true for a man that it is more pleasurable when he feels his partner contracting her vaginal muscles during intercourse.

The lower part of the vagina is surrounded by a muscular ring, which forms part of the pelvic-floor muscle. Most women are encouraged to carry out pelvic-floor exercises after childbirth to encourage the muscle to resume its normal tone. However, after a difficult labour and birth, or a large baby, some or all of the muscle fibres may be torn and the normal constricting function may be lost, resulting in the condition known as 'lax vagina'. The operation to correct this is medically known as a posterior repair. Gynaecologists as well as cosmetic surgeons perform it. The more common anterior repair is done by gynaecologists for stress incontinence and prolapse of the uterus.

At consultation, the surgeon needs to ensure that this is truly a case of lax vagina and that the symptoms are not due to psychosexual problems for which surgery is unhelpful. The simple test is to place two fingers inside the vagina and ask the woman to grip them as tightly as possible. If the increase in pressure is feeble or absent altogether, then it is likely that repairing the muscle will be effective. If there is strong muscle tone then surgery has little to offer.

The operation

You will be admitted on the morning of the operation and a general anaesthetic is given (see pages 61–63). You will be placed on the operating table lying on your back with your legs lifted apart in what is referred to as the 'lithotomy' position. A vertical incision is made in the lining of the vagina, internally, and this lining layer is undermined to expose the underlying muscle layer. The muscles are appropriately tightened with stitches taking great care not to damage the rectum, which is situated immediately behind. The excess lining is trimmed and the incision sutured with dissolvable stitches. A small paraffin gauze tampon is placed inside the vagina to exert some counter pressure. This reduces bleeding and swelling and encourages the skin to stick to the muscles in their new position. Most patients stay overnight for observation.

Postoperative events

Bleeding Many patients may experience a slight ooze from the incision line for a day or two. The tampon is removed the following day, but if bleeding continues another tampon can be inserted until it stops.

Pain There will be a dragging soreness for a few days with sharp pains on coughing, lifting or any activity that causes the tummy muscles to contract.

Urinary retention Swelling in the vagina can affect the urethra, the urinary outflow tube, and possibly cause it to obstruct. It is important that your clinic ensures that you can urinate normally before you are discharged.

Sexual intercourse This can usually be resumed about three weeks after the operation, but not before any soreness or discharge has settled. It should be started cautiously, and stopped if there is any discomfort. A vaginal lubricant may be helpful initially until all discomfort ceases.

Infection This is an uncommon occurrence and would cause a discharge. If the discharge persists for more than a few days it should be investigated further by your surgeon to exclude an infection.

Result
In cases of genuine lax vagina this procedure is very successful, with patients reporting much more satisfactory lovemaking that is also appreciated by their partners.

HYMEN REPAIR

In those societies where virginity is highly prized, some women find themselves in a difficult and embarrassing situation. It is possible to insert an absorbable suture around the opening of the vagina and repair tears in the hymen if any of it remains. This gives quite a realistic impression of virginity.

G-SPOT IMPLANT AND LABIAL IMPLANTS

The G-spot is a small area of very sensitive tissue on the front wall of the vagina about 2cm (1in) in from the opening. It is claimed that friction with this tissue during intercourse brings about vaginal orgasm. Injection of filler material into this area makes it project more and thus facilitates greater friction with the penis during intercourse. Filler can also be injected around the opening of the vagina, called the introitus, increasing the sensations of both partners.

As a woman ages, the outer vulval lips can reduce in size. If this presents a problem, the patient's own fat can be implanted in the vulval lips to provide a satisfactory solution.

VULVAPLASTY

There is a very wide variation in what is considered normal in a vulva. There are two sets of lips. The outer lips are bulky and fold round from the front to meet at the back. The inner ones are much thinner and meet at the front to form the hood of the clitoris. In infants the inner lips don't usually protrude at all, but after puberty they grow in size and project past the outer lips a short distance in most women.

Sometimes the inner lips are quite large and bulky. Although they are entirely normal if they are like this, some women are embarrassed by them because they show as a lump in underclothes or swimwear and they can chafe and become sore. There are various procedures that aim to trim them back so that the vulva looks neater.

It is important that the surgeon does not trim away the sensitive tissue near the clitoris. The operation is quite simple and can be done as a day case. Afterwards the area is very sensitive for a few days and it may be several weeks before sexual intercourse can be resumed.

CLITORAL REDUCTION

Some women have an unusually large clitoris, either as a result of a developmental anomaly or taking steroids. It can be reduced effectively by dissecting out the shaft (the structure of the clitoris is like a tiny penis), trimming it as necessary and then sewing the head of the clitoris onto the base. This technique if done carefully should not affect the all-important sensitivity.

MONS REDUCTION

Some women have a very prominent *mons veneris* that shows in underclothes and swimwear and even produces a bump in sheer dresses. It can be satisfactorily reduced by liposuction in most cases.

Vascular Cosmetic Surgery

VARICOSE VEINS

Varicose veins are abnormal, tortuous (snake like), dilated superficial veins that usually affect the legs. They occur in about 20 per cent of the population in the UK. The incidence increases with age and is equally distributed between the sexes, although fives times as many women as men go to their GP about it. This condition, together with its associated complications, accounts for approximately half a million GP consultations in the UK every year.

In about 40 per cent of cases, the condition is inherited and there are often no obvious predisposing factors, the commonest of which are obesity, pregnancy, oral contraceptives, hormone-replacement therapy and excessive standing.

In many cases, sufferers wait until the condition has become very widespread and unsightly or is causing symptoms of pain and discomfort, before seeking treatment. In some cases help is only sought when a 'venous ulcer' (one that is not responding to standard treatment or has become infected) has developed – usually around the ankle area.

How Varicose Veins Develop

In order to understand how varicose veins develop in the first instance a simple explanation and basic understanding of the venous anatomy of the leg is required. There are two systems of venous drainage in the leg: the superficial and the deep. It is important to appreciate that all healthy leg veins have one-way valves, which enhance blood flow back to the heart. During walking or other active movements of the leg muscles, the veins are squeezed and emptied. When the muscles relax the veins fill again.

Regular contracting and relaxation of the leg muscles, aided by the one-way valves, actively pumps the venous blood back to the heart. When standing the muscles are relaxed. This makes the veins distend and if they become stretched the valves may not work properly.

The two systems are connected by one-way valves so that in the normal situation blood can flow from the superficial to the deep system, either directly as at the groin and back of the knee, or through perforator veins. Perforator veins are specific veins, guarded by one-way valves, designed to connect the superficial and deep systems, piercing or perforating the deep tissues to constitute a connection at various sites in the lower leg and thigh.

The vast majority (95 per cent) of varicose veins (Primary varicose veins) are caused by an increase in venous pressure in the superficial leg veins due to damage to the valves in the perforator veins that connect the superficial to the deep venous systems. The little one-way valves in the leg veins gradually become damaged and incompetent (leak) causing a build-up of pressure in the vein. This build-up of pressure damages the next valve below. Gradually more and more valves will be damaged and the condition slowly worsens as the veins become more dilated, tortuous and increasingly more prominent.

Symptoms include aching, itching, throbbing and ankle swelling. Complications include spontaneous bleeding, inflammation (thrombophlebitis), skin changes e.g. inflammatory changes (lipodermatosclerosis), pigmentation, ulceration and eczema. Treatment will depend on the severity of each case and will be largely governed by the patient's attitude towards the cosmetic appearance as well as any symptoms or complications.

Investigations

Before treatment is undertaken it is important to perform investigations in order to establish two facts:

1. The sites where there is a leak between the two systems of veins.
2. Whether the deep system is patent, especially in those who have previously suffered a deep vein thrombosis. In other words to exclude a complete or partial blockage of the deep system. This is necessary, as removing superficial varicose veins in this situation will worsen the pressure in the superficial system and lead to a rapid recurrence of varicose veins.

Treatments

There are several different treatment methods available.

Compression Stockings

This method has a limited role in selected cases to control symptoms. It does not reduce or rid the legs of the diseased veins, and many people find them unsightly. To have any worthwhile effect they must be worn continuously when not in bed. They are recommended for those who have to stand a lot because they can be beneficial in preventing a worsening of the condition.

Sclerotherapy

This technique was once the mainstay of treatment of varicose veins in the UK. It is rapidly being superseded by other techniques, which are more reliable and successful.

This treatment involves the injection of selected varicose veins with a sclerosant solution. A sclerosant is a chemical that causes an inflammation of the lining of the vein wall. Using compression bandages on the legs after injection, the vein walls are pushed together. The inflammation of the lining of the vein wall causes the walls to stick together, thereby blocking and closing the vein. This effectively makes the vein disappear, as blood will no longer flow through it, although a hard cord can remain for several weeks before it finally resolves. This hard cord is the result of the inflammation of the lining of the vein wall (thrombophlebitis), which can cause pain and discomfort.

After a course of injections, patients are encouraged to walk several miles daily for several weeks in an attempt to prevent a deep vein thrombosis (DVT) in the event that the sclerosant solution entered the deep venous system through an incompetent perforating vein.

Pain and discomfort, wearing bandages constantly for several weeks and walking several miles daily makes this an unpleasant treatment for the majority of patients. Coupled with a 70 per cent or higher recurrence rate within five years it is not hard to appreciate the reasons for the decline in popularity of this treatment when more modern, successful and easily tolerated treatments with less recovery time are available.

Foam sclerotherapy

There has recently been a resurgence of interest in sclerotherapy using a slightly modified technique that was first introduced in 1944 but which fell out of favour over the years. The technique involves injecting foam, produced by mixing sclerosant fluid with air, under ultrasound guidance into the affected vein. Results using this technique are encouraging and research is ongoing. Some senior surgeons are actively promoting this technique as they are getting excellent results.

Surgery

Those cases that do not have a leaking valve in the groin (at the junction where the main superficial vein drains into the deep vein of the leg) can be treated on a day-care basis. Those cases with a leaking valve in the groin vein require more extensive surgery. The procedure is called a phlebectomy or multiple avulsions (stripping out) of varicose veins. It is usually performed under general anaesthetic and one or more night's stay in the clinic will be necessary. Some surgeons do however perform this operation on a day-care basis under local anaesthetic.

Cases suitable for day care surgery

You will be admitted to the clinic on the morning of the surgery. The veins are marked out on the skin surface while you are standing. The sites of incompetent (leaking) perforating veins are also marked.

You will then be taken to theatre and sedated with an intravenous injection. The area to be operated on is then anaesthetised with local anaesthetic. Once the anaesthetic has taken effect, tiny stab incisions are made over the varicose veins and they are removed piece by piece by pulling them away from the tissues under the skin, with special instruments. The end of the vein is not tied off, as a compression bandage will shut the vein at the end of the operation until it heals and shuts off permanently.

Because the incisions are tiny, sutures are unnecessary. Special attention is paid to the sites where a perforating vein with an incompetent (leaking) valve is present. This perforating vein is located and divided (cut), and each end is closed by tying a knot of suture material around it.

On completion of the operation, dressings and a pressure bandage are applied for one week. You will usually be discharged home about an hour after surgery and given postoperative instructions. You will be forbidden to drive initially, so must arrange for suitable transport to take you home.

Cases with a leaking valve in the groin

You will be admitted to the clinic on the morning of surgery. A general anaesthetic is usually administered although many surgeons now perform the procedure under sedation and local anaesthetic. The varicose veins are removed as described above. In addition, the valve in the groin vein is tied off through a small incision in the groin. Likewise the superficial vein entering the deep vein at the back of the knee is tied off at the junction of the two. The stay in the clinic is usually no longer than one day.

Postoperative events

Bleeding This is most likely to occur in the immediate postoperative period. Local pressure and elevation of the leg is all that is required.

Pain and discomfort This is uncommon and if it occurs it only lasts for a short time. Painkillers are usually prescribed.

Scars The tiny scars in the legs are usually barely noticeable once they have matured after a few weeks.

Bruising and swelling This occurs in varying degrees and usually resolves within a few days.

Discolouration Very rarely the bruising does not resolve completely, leaving purple or blue discolouration. The reasons for this are not clear and the condition can be permanent.

Spider veins In a small number of cases spider or thread veins can appear. It is impossible to predict with any degree of accuracy which patients will develop this complication, although those who already have areas of spider veins do seem to be more likely to suffer this effect. There are now newer and successful methods of treating these thread veins (see below, page 189).

Nerve damage (neuropraxia) Occasionally a superficial sensory nerve can be damaged, resulting in a decrease in or loss of sensation as well as discomfort in an area. These symptoms resolve once the nerve has regenerated (healed).

Recurrence It must be firmly understood that those diseased veins which have been removed cannot recur. Those who have a tendency or predisposition to form varicose veins have a 20-per-cent chance of developing further varicose veins within five years.

Postoperative management

The leg should be elevated as much as possible for the first 24 hours. Sleeping with the leg elevated for the first night is also recommended. Sometimes the bandage will feel too tight and will need to be reapplied. If bleeding occurs through the bandage, rest and elevation of the leg is necessary and another bandage may have to be applied. Full mobilisation is usually permitted after the first 24 to 48 hours.

Laser Treatment

Endo venous laser treatment is a relatively new procedure in the UK that is rapidly gaining popularity for many reasons: it is less invasive; can be performed under local anaesthetic on a day-care basis; has a short operation time; and a rapid recovery with reduced postoperative discomfort or pain. It is considered by many authorities that within the next few years this technique will supersede current open surgical vein-stripping procedures (see above).

Technique

Under local anaesthetic a small incision is made over the offending diseased varicose vein and a thin laser catheter is inserted into it and passed under ultrasound control to the valve at the groin. The heat produced from the laser catheter as it is being withdrawn induces an 'in situ' thrombosis, which shuts off the vein permanently. The procedure only takes a few minutes and discomfort is minimal.

Aftercare and results

Afterwards the incision is dressed and after a short recovery period most patients are allowed home. Full recovery generally takes about a fortnight. Postoperative bruising, swelling, pain and discomfort are minimal, and most patients are able to return to work within 24 hours.

The long-term results of this technique are still being evaluated but preliminary results in most centres are very encouraging.

SPIDER OR THREAD VEINS

Thread veins are abnormally dilated (widened), small blood vessels very close to the surface of the skin. They most commonly occur on the face and legs. The tendency to them is usually inherited. They become more prominent with increasing age and can occur in clusters, especially on the face, causing patchy discolouration (redness).

Thread veins are worsened by excessive exposure to the sun and wind and extremes of temperature. Alcohol consumption causes thread veins to become more dilated and thus makes them even more prominent.

In those who are predisposed to this irritating condition, it should be mentioned that any treatment of varicose veins, i.e. by injections or surgery, could exacerbate the appearance of thread veins in the legs (see above).

Finally it must always be appreciated that this is an ongoing condition and either the spider veins recur or new ones appear. No treatment is therefore permanent.

Treatment

Recent years have seen an increasing number of different treatments available for this irritating problem. The mainstay at present still seems to be injection sclerotherapy (see above), but newer treatments e.g. thermo-coagulation, intense pulsed light and laser technology are becoming more popular. At this time it is not possible to predict which method will be the mainstay of treatment in the future.

Some schools of thought do not advocate using microsclerotherapy for treating spider veins on the face, because of the risk of scarring or pigment changes, which to many women will be unacceptable. Others will happily advocate this treatment, as it is generally very successful especially if performed by an expert. Injection microsclerotherapy is particularly successful on the legs, but treatment must be performed by a practitioner who specialises in this technique and performs it on a frequent basis. It takes great skill and practice to introduce a needle into a thin narrow vein without damaging it. The main drawback of this technique is that several sessions are required in the majority of cases in order to achieve a worthwhile result. The main advantage is that the cost is generally lower than using other more sophisticated techniques.

Although the current lasers can cause pigmentation changes, especially when used on the legs, newer ones are constantly being introduced which reduce this unwanted effect.

It must also be appreciated that practitioners who specialise in the treatment of spider veins will adopt their own chosen technique that gives them the best results e.g. some may be adept at microsclerotherapy, and get excellent results with the minimum of complications. Others may not be as good and may even have abandoned this technique for an easier option using a device which, although costly, gives them better results. As a result, different practitioners will claim that their technique is better so there is no universally accepted method, which can be claimed to be superior.

Many different types of practitioner, from beauty therapists to surgeons, can treat thread veins successfully in all sorts of ways. A simple technique done by a beautician in the High Street can be just as effective as advanced laser treatment carried out in a swish clinic – and it can be much more convenient and less expensive.

Injection Microsclerotherapy

This method is more suitable for the larger thread veins in the legs. The treatment is uncomfortable, but not painful and is performed on an outpatient basis. Sclerosing fluid (see above) is injected directly into the thread vein using a very fine needle. The inflammation produced causes the walls of the vessel to stick together thereby preventing blood flow through it and thus making it invisible. Several injection sessions at two- to four-weekly intervals may be necessary, and recurrence is common. Heavy-duty elastic compression stockings (tights) should be worn for a few days afterwards.

Postoperative events

Bruising Localised bruising, swelling and redness is common initially and this usually resolves within a few days but can take a lot longer.

Discolouration On rare occasions a red or brown discolouration may occur at the injection site. This may take several months to fade but can be permanent.

Matting A complication known as 'matting' can sometimes occur temporarily following microsclerotherapy. This occurs when fine, red veins appear as a result of new blood vessels being formed (angiogenesis) or as a result of the dilatation of existing veins that were previously invisible. The appearance can range from a network of fine red veins to a patchy red discolouration, which blanches on pressure. Thankfully this condition usually resolves by itself over three to six months. Rarely it can be permanent, but treatment by laser has been shown to be successful.

Ulceration On rare occasions, a small area of ulceration can occur over an injection site resulting in a scar, which will usually fade in time. On very rare occasions, thrombophlebitis (inflammation of the superficial veins) (see page 186) and pulmonary embolus (clot in the lung) (see page 40) have been reported.

Thermo-Coagulation

The technique of thermo-coagulation employs high-frequency microwave energy to heat and thus destroy the offending thread veins, resulting in their complete disappearance. A very fine insulated needle is introduced just under the skin surface close to the offending thread vein. A current is passed, which destroys the thread vein. The surrounding skin and tissue is protected and preserved without damage.

Treatment is performed with the minimum of discomfort on a walk-in, walk-out basis. No bandages or support tights are required afterwards. There is usually no bruising although some redness may persist for a few days. Normal activities can be resumed immediately after treatment.

This technique can be used on all skin types, as there is no loss of skin pigmentation afterwards, and on any part of the body. Since its introduction, this technique has extended its use to improve the results of microsclerotherapy (see above) as well as treating other skin conditions.

Laser Treatment

Lasers (see pages 119–122 for more detailed information about lasers) work by firing powerful, short bursts of light energy on the thread vein causing it to collapse. With no blood flowing through it, the vein will no longer be visible.

Laser technology is constantly being developed and newer lasers for treating thread veins on the face and legs appear regularly. Patients can walk into the treatment room, have it done and walk out again. The treatment is not usually painful. Transient redness over the treated area is common. Some lasers cause hypo-pigmentation (skin becomes lighter in colour) over the treated area, which can take a long time to resolve.

Intense Pulsed Light (IPL)

(See pages 122–123 for more detailed information about IPL.) This method uses short pulses of light energy to coagulate (clot) the blood in the thread vein causing it to disappear. This non-invasive technique can be used on the face and legs and is suitable for all skin types and colours. Treatment is performed on a walk-in, walk-out basis with minimum discomfort. Any reddening of the skin afterwards will disappear after a few minutes.

Removal of Tattoos

Tattoos are probably one of the oldest forms of body decoration, with a history stretching back to the Stone Age. Tattooing is the introduction of pigment into the deep layer of the skin to produce a permanent mark. It may occur sometimes as a result of an accident when dark coloured material is implanted into a wound. Occasionally such traumatic tattooing can be extensive, especially after an abrasive wound, and these should be treated at the time of injury by vigorous scrubbing of the abraded area.

Decorative tattoos are either self-inflicted or professionally performed. Professional tattoos are made up of clumps of pigmented carbon particles, which are injected into the deep layer of the skin. The carbon particles are too large to be removed and excreted by the body's own immune system. Instead the body isolates itself from these invading particles by forming a protective layer of scar tissue around them.

Recent fashion trends have inspired more women to have tattoos printed on various parts of their body and many are quite proud to show them off. Only time will tell if this trend will continue and whether they will one day regret their decision. Fashions change but tattoos don't, and often they look inappropriate many years later.

Unfortunately it is a lot more difficult to remove a tattoo than to apply it the first place, and more expensive. The regretted tattoo can be removed, but only at the expense of significant scarring in many cases. There are several treatment options.

Excision with or without a skin graft

A small tattoo can be totally excised (cut out) and the resulting wound closed with stitches. If the tattoo is large it may be excised and the resulting defect covered with a skin graft if the skin edges cannot be brought together and sutured. The result is usually preferable to the original tattoo but there will always be a scar.

Lasers

Lasers are devices that produce a powerful controlled beam of light energy in short bursts (pulses). The energy from this light beam is absorbed by a specific colour only (not by the surrounding tissue) and thermal (heat) energy is produced. At low power a localised burn is produced. At high power the targeted cells are instantly vaporised.

When the laser is aimed at a tattoo, the energy is absorbed by the colour in the pigmented particles of the tattoo, resulting in the particles being broken down into smaller, minute particles, which can then be absorbed and excreted by the body. This process is called 'phagocytosis'. Green, yellow and purple are harder to remove than black or red.

The Nd:YAG and Ruby Q-Switched lasers (see page 119) are the lasers most commonly used to remove professional tattoos. The number of treatments required to remove a tattoo will depend on the type, depth and age of the tattoo, the skin's reaction to laser light and the presence of any existing skin conditions. Usually a gradual fading occurs after every treatment.

Treatment is performed on an outpatient basis and usually produces only a mild discomfort so that local anaesthesia is rarely needed. Redness and flushing can last up to six or eight weeks and further treatment is withheld until this has fully resolved. Scarring can occur if the power setting on the laser is set too high.

When the Yag laser is used the treated area is covered in white marks and pinpoint bleeding may occur. A small amount of scabbing will appear in the first week. The skin may then become dry and pink before it fully heals.

When the Ruby laser is used swelling may occur and occasionally blisters will form. The area may become itchy for a while.

Laser tattoo removal is now the treatment of choice in most cases and more sophisticated lasers are being developed to deal with the more difficult colours.

Postoperative events

Where a tattoo has been excised and the defect sutured the resulting scar may become stretched or thickened depending on the site of excision and the tension under which it was sutured.

Where a skin graft has been used there will always be a permanent mark. The grafted area will be hairless and a different colour compared to the surrounding skin. Altered pigmentation as a result of sunburn may occur and the margins of the graft may become red and raised.

Improving Unsightly Scars

Unsightly scars and blemishes can very often be improved by well-planned and carefully executed surgery. It must be stressed that no cosmetic surgeon can produce invisible scars. He can only make the scars as inconspicuous as possible. The aim of scar revision is to achieve a scar that is fine, level and even with the surrounding tissue, about the same colour as the adjacent skin and that causes no pull on the surrounding structures. These are the optimum conditions that will make a scar less visible or noticeable to the observer, but it will not be invisible.

It can take six to 18 months for any scar to mature, at which point little or no further change or improvement will occur. Initially any scar will be red and raised above the level of the surrounding skin and may often be hard in consistency. Gradually the redness and hardness lessen and resolve, leaving a soft scar that is level with and somewhat paler than the adjacent skin.

For this reason scar revision must not be undertaken too soon because adequate time must elapse to allow the healing tissues to mature.

If there is tension across the edges of a wound as it is healing, the resulting scar will be wide, because the skin edges pull apart during healing. All skin has a slight natural tension in all directions, but in nearly all areas of the body this tension is much greater in one direction than another at right angles to it. This means that if two incisions are made close to each other in the same area of skin, but one incision is lined up to be parallel to the strongest tension and the other is at right angles to the first, the incision that is parallel to the tension will produce a much better scar.

Elective surgical incisions are placed as far as possible to be parallel to skin tension, whereas wounds obviously tend to be more randomly orientated. This is why a surgical scar should heal more neatly than one caused by an injury. In carrying out scar revision the surgeon will do his best to change the orientation of the scar so that it is optimum. This is why scar revisions often include strange shapes such as Z or W. Indeed changing a stretched linear scar into a Z shape, called a Z-plasty is a very frequent plastic surgery operation.

Apart from becoming wide or lumpy, some scars can become deeply dented, because the fat layer is missing and the skin becomes attached to the deep layers of body tissue instead of smoothly sliding over them, which is the usual situation. Appendicectomy scars are especially prone to this. Scar revision in such cases involves lifting the skin away from the deep tissue layers, re-establishing the fat layer and finally tidying up the skin scar.

Some areas of the body always produce noticeable scars e.g. nose, chin, chest, shoulders, upper back and parts of the arms and legs.

In summary therefore, the goal in scar revision is improvement and not perfection. A scar cannot be made to vanish into thin air.

The operation

You will be admitted on the morning of surgery. Most facial scars can be revised under local anaesthesia. Extensive scarring in adults and scars in children are best treated under general anaesthetic. Most scar-revision procedures can be treated on a day-care basis but some may require an overnight stay in the clinic.

The old unsightly scar has to be removed first. Any planned surgical incision heals in exactly the same manner as any other deliberate or accidental cut, i.e. it produces scar tissue, which is nature's method of healing. Once an incision is made and sutured the surgeon has little control over the healing process, a fact that must be appreciated by the patient.

When revising a scar on the face the surgeon attempts to get the best possible result by placing the new scars parallel to or actually in one of the normal crease lines of the face. This usually means that the direction and shape of the original scar may have to be changed.

Excision of large scars or blemishes may require several operations over a period of time.

Postoperative events

Unfavourable results will still occur when a scar becomes stretched, thickened or infected even after a carefully executed and timed revision procedure. Even in the best of cases, the original scar will only have been improved, not vanished altogether.

Non-Surgical Treatments

In many instances, if a scar is still unsightly once it has fully matured and no further improvement will occur naturally, other methods of improvement are available besides the type of surgery described above.

Raised scars

Steroid injections are used initially in hypertrophic or keloid (raised and thickened) scars to reduce their size and projection down to the level of the surrounding skin. Scars that end up being raised as a bump above the surrounding skin can be planed down with a laser (see pages 119–122 and page 195), dermabrasion (see pages 110–113) or chemical peel (see pages 113–115). This will make the scar less conspicuous to the observer and easier to disguise with make-up.

Colour changes

Some scars end up looking redder than the surrounding skin as the result of an increased number of blood vessels in them. In the darker or black-skinned individual, the scar may end up looking darker or lighter than the surrounding skin. This makes the scar much more noticeable.

Where the scar is more conspicuous as a result of an increase in the number of blood vessels or pigment, improvement can be obtained using a laser (see pages 119–122 and page 195). The laser can reduce the number of blood vessels in the scar as well as the amount of pigment in it, thus making the scar more compatible with the colour of the surrounding skin.

A laser cannot add pigment to a scar that is lighter in colour than the surrounding skin. In this situation colour can be added to the scar using a method similar to tattooing where a coloured pigment of the same colour as the surrounding skin is injected into the scar.

Acne scarring

Acne scarring can be treated in a number of ways depending on the type, distribution and size of the scars. A large area full of depressed scars responds well to laser resurfacing (see pages 119–122), dermabrasion (see pages 110–113) or chemical peeling (see pages 113–115). Several sessions may be required to obtain the optimum aesthetic appearance.

So-called 'ice-pick scars' (deep holes) respond best to excision (cutting them out) and suturing the skin edges together. Alternatively a 'cylindrical punch' instrument can be used to cut out the scar and replace the defect with a cylindrical piece of skin cut from behind the ear.

Fillers

Dermal fillers (see pages 101–109) have a limited use in depressed scars on the face. The result is usually temporary and regular top-up injections are required. Nevertheless, a small group of suitable patients elect to undergo this method.

Results

It is most unlikely that any scar can be removed completely, and become invisible. The aim of the procedure is to make a scar less noticeable and perhaps easier to disguise with make-up. We hope that in the not too distant future, new technology will enable us to produce invisible scars.

The Treatment of Hair Loss

Hair loss can be a particularly unpleasant and embarrassing experience for women. Temporary hair loss can be caused by illness (e.g. thyroid disorders), various medicines (including chemotherapy for cancer treatment), infections and psychological causes arising from acute trauma to long-term stress. Permanent hair loss is usually the result of genetic factors associated with hormonal imbalance.

Temporary hair loss is usually remedied easily once the direct cause or the predisposing factors have been determined and brought under control. Hair growth will then return to its normal pattern.

Permanent hair loss can only be effectively treated by surgery. Surgery cannot give a bald person more hair. However, the remaining hair (at the back and sides of the scalp) can be surgically repositioned to give an aesthetically pleasing hair cover in suitable cases, provided that treatment is performed by experts in the field.

Not everyone is suitable for surgery and each case must be carefully evaluated before a treatment programme is started. Every patient who contemplates embarking on a treatment programme must ensure that she is properly advised by an expert and fully understands the nature of the treatment, as well as the probable outcome and limitations.

Although hair replacement surgery is predominantly performed in males, the hair transplant surgeon is seeing more women seeking this treatment. Current trends show that about 10 per cent of a hair transplant surgeon's clientele is female and this percentage is rising.

In recent years topical preparations (medicines directly applied to the scalp) have been successfully used to effectively halt the process of hair loss in women and these are discussed more fully below. Some women will experience a temporary substantial hair loss for no apparent reason and, unlike this kind of hair loss in men, hair will eventually re-grow without resorting to any treatment.

Hair Loss in Women

Very few things will devastate a woman's self esteem more than losing her hair. Thinning hair in a woman is perceived as a loss of beauty and can go on to adversely affect her personal and professional life.

Hair loss is surprisingly common in women, despite the fact that many women suffering from this condition will not often appear in public without attempting to hide their problem, usually by wearing a wig or head scarf.

In most cases, hair loss in women is genetically determined, and about one in four suffer from thinning hair as a result of androgenic (male hormone) alopecia or 'female pattern baldness'. All women have male as well as female hormones in their system. Male pattern baldness is caused by a gene, which converts large quantities of testosterone (male hormone) to dihydrotestosterone or DHT, which damages the hair follicle. A scalp hair follicle has a life cycle of approximately five years. For four of the five years the follicle is in the growing phase and in the last year it becomes dormant. Follicles that become damaged as a result of the adverse effects of DHT fall out and are not replaced. Reduction of female hormone or an overproduction of male hormone will permit the dominant male hormone to exert its adverse effects on the hair follicles, causing the hair to fall out.

In women, unlike in the majority of men, the hair loss pattern is somewhat different. Typically a generalised loss or thinning occurs over the entire scalp; or, the hairline remains intact with significant thinning beginning behind the hairline and extending to the crown. Fortunately in most cases this thinning does not progress to total baldness.

The onset of hair loss can begin as early as the late teens but most commonly occurs just before or during the menopause – a time of hormonal flux when the protective female hormonal levels decline. Other causes of hair loss are attributed to drugs and psychological events, which can lead to a reduction in circulating female hormones. The commonest cause of a receding hairline in women is facelifting (see pages 74–84).

This condition is now eminently treatable, with current state-of-the-art technology and the expertise of dedicated hair-transplant surgeons. Hair-follicle grafts can now be safely and successfully transplanted into the thinning area by interspersing them between existing hair follicles. This results in an overall increase in hair density without damaging the existing hair follicles.

Preoperative assessment

A hair-transplant surgeon has to take the following into account before advising on the most suitable treatment programme for you.

• Your age and the amount of current hair loss.
• The probable future loss of hair.
• The quality and quantity of donor hair available.
• Your expectations.

It is now universally accepted by hair-transplant surgeons that meticulous preoperative planning is of paramount importance in order to achieve the best possible results. Probable future hair loss has to be seriously considered so that there will be enough donor hair left to cater for future hair loss. The initial positioning of the hairline has to be conservative for the same reasons.

At the preoperative assessment the procedure must be fully explained. Of utmost importance to consider are the likely result and your expectations. This is particularly important because hair transplantation usually entails a series of procedures spaced out at intervals of a minimum of three to four months. The number of procedures is individually tailored according to requirements but usually two to three procedures are performed on average in each patient.

Hair-transplant technology has escalated in recent years leading to far more natural and successful results. In addition, a better understanding of hair physiology has enabled the skilfully executed hair transplant to obtain a much better yield of hair growth from each transplanted graft.

Follicular units

Hair grows in small units referred to as 'follicular units'. A follicular unit consists of one to four hair follicles. It also contains oil glands, a small muscle (to make the hair stand on end) and tiny nerves and blood vessels. A follicular unit is a hair-bearing component of skin, which must be kept intact in order to ensure maximum hair growth when it is transplanted to another site in the scalp.

Current trends

The current thinking by most hair-transplant surgeons is to give priority to transplanting hair follicles to the frontal scalp and not to transplant the crown. In this way, all available donor hair is utilised in the most efficient manner to give the best long-term result. It must be emphasised, however, that every case is treated on its own merits after a detailed consultation with the operating surgeon. The reason behind this thinking is that most people who look at themselves in a mirror will not be able to see the back of their scalp hence not be frequently reminded of their hair loss there.

SURGICAL PROCEDURES

Hair Transplantation

Prior to any invasive manoeuvre, the surgeon marks out the proposed hairline and area to be grafted. The position of the proposed hairline will depend on the individual situation after a detailed discussion with the patient. The donor site at the back of the scalp is shaved and surrounding hair pinned back to give the surgeon full access to harvest the donor hair.

Under sedation and local anaesthetic, a strip of hair-bearing scalp, approximately 1cm wide and between 5 and 25 cm long, is cut from the back of the scalp. The incision is then sutured with dissolvable stitches. The resulting scar is adequately covered by the surrounding hair.

The next important step is to carefully cut the donor strip into miniature slivers, which are then meticulously segmented into follicular units (see above) under the extreme magnification of a stereoscopic microscope. Care is especially taken to avoid damage to adjacent hairs, oil glands and hair roots.

Once all the grafts have been prepared, tiny slits are made in the hairline and recipient area of the scalp. The angle and direction of the slits are important in order to mimic the natural hairline and growth pattern. Each graft is then inserted into the prepared slit. No dressing or bandage is applied as this will invariably dislodge or pull out some of the grafts on removal.

The patient is then sent to the recovery room to sleep off the sedative before being checked over by the surgeon and finally allowed home. Painkillers and sedatives are usually given to take home, as well as a short course of low-dose steroid tablets to minimise postoperative swelling.

The entire procedure takes between two and five hours depending on the speed of the team and the amount of work required per patient.

The bandage and dressing is removed the following day and the hair is gently washed. The next procedure cannot be carried out for another four months or until the hair starts to grow from the previous procedure. This is because the surgeon needs to be fully aware of where to transplant the next set of grafts and not damage any existing hair follicles.

Postoperative events

In the first three weeks following surgical hair transplantation, the transplanted hair will appear to be growing quickly. In reality the follicle is in a dormant state, attempting to recover from the traumatic experience of the operation. As a result, many but not all these hairs will fall out. After a period of recovery the follicle will yield a new hair, which will take between 12 and 14 weeks to appear through the scalp surface and continue to grow as normal.

Pain Mild to moderate discomfort is usually experienced with hair transplantation. Oral painkillers are usually prescribed.

Bruising and swelling This often occurs around the eyes. It can last a few days and is not usually severe. Adequate postoperative medication can reduce or even prevent this undesirable complication.

Bleeding Bleeding following this procedure is extremely rare. If it does occur it responds to simple pressure. Sometimes the bandage will have to be applied again for 24 hours to help stop the bleeding.

Itching The scalp is often itchy but this is rarely troublesome.

Infection This complication is rare. Antibiotics are routinely prescribed during the postoperative period.

Numbness Some transient numbness of the scalp may occur. If it occurs it can last a few months. Usually you will not even notice it.

Scabbing and scarring After transplantation, scabs will form on the transplanted units, which fall off after a few weeks. Some hairs may fall out together with the scabs but these will re-grow in about three months. The scars are visible for a while but will fade in time. The surrounding hair covers the donor scar. Occasionally the donor scar can stretch and become visible, especially if the hair is cut very short. A scar revision may then be necessary (see 'Improving Unsightly Scars', pages 196–199).

Sudden loss of hair in the transplanted area (anagen effluvium) On rare occasions there may be a sudden loss of existing hair occurring in the transplanted area about two months after surgery. This can be very distressing for the patient and reassurance by the surgeon at the time is very important. The cause is unknown but is thought to be related to the trauma of the initial surgery. In nearly all cases the hair will eventually grow back.

Most surgeons feel that the incidence of this complication is reduced by the topical application of Minoxidil (see below) before and after surgery.

Failure of hair growth   The failure of hair to grow can occur as a result of poor surgical technique or infection. On rare occasions there is no apparent cause.

Results

It is certainly true to say that a poor hair transplant looks unsightly and attracts more attention than the original hair loss. Nowadays, however, with proper patient selection and expert treatment a very pleasing result can usually be achieved.

Using modern hair transplant techniques, most patients can be helped. However those who are not ideal candidates must have realistic expectations. The hair-transplant surgeon is limited by the amount of donor hair at his disposal, and has to take into account unpredictable future hair loss.

Using micro-grafting techniques, other areas such as the eyebrows and eyelashes can be successfully treated. In addition more women are having hair transplantation to the scars in the temples following a face lift.

It must be emphasised that although the technique of hair transplantation may appear technically simple, in reality it takes many years of experience and dedication to produce consistently good results. Prospective patients are therefore advised to take great care in selecting their hair-transplant surgeon. Nowadays all reputable hair transplant surgeons will be able to produce appropriate certificates and proof of training in their field.

NON-SURGICAL TREATMENTS

There have been innumerable claims over the years to cure hair loss in women and none of these have been shown to be effective to date except for Minoxidil. Indeed, we warn any woman suffering from hair loss to beware of any media advertising that claims to offer a cure or worthwhile treatment for hair loss, without seeking proper medical advice, as invariably these claims prove to be a money making scam.

Minoxidil (Regaine®)

Minoxidil is a drug originally used to control blood pressure. It was soon discovered that it promoted hair growth. It is applied to the scalp as a topical solution.

It is believed to act by reversing the genetic process of hair follicle shrinkage. To this effect it must be applied twice daily indefinitely to achieve a worthwhile result. In some cases it can cause scalp irritation but if it is discontinued any hair that has been retained or saved will fall out.

It is available as a lotion in two and five per cent concentrations.

HAIR REMOVAL

Unwanted body hair is an extremely common problem. There are various methods of hair removal from simple home remedies such as shaving, plucking, waxing, depilatory creams etc. to more sophisticated and scientific techniques, which offer a more long lasting effect e.g. intense pulsed light (IPL) (see pages 122–123, and below), or lasers (see pages 119–122, and below).

Body-hair distribution is genetically unique to every individual and race e.g. excessive facial hair growth in women (hirsutism) can be normal (genetic) or be associated with a variety of medical disorders. Menopausal women are often troubled by hair on the face. This is due to the high levels of androgenic (masculinising) hormones produced by their bodies at that time. Most women are very reluctant to start shaving and thus seek permanent methods of hair removal.

It is fair to say that most practitioners who specialise in hair removal will use a technique that is simple to administer, gives successful results and has few problems. It must be added that technology is constantly being improved and newer devices for hair removal are constantly being developed. However, the cost of many of these new devices may be prohibitive to many practitioners, resulting in the prospective patient not necessarily being offered the most up-to-date and successful treatment options.

The Normal Hair-Growth Cycle

In order to understand how hair removal works it is necessary to know how a normal hair develops and grows. Each hair is made up of a shaft (the part visible above the skin surface) and a root (the part buried under the skin). At the end of the root is a swelling called a hair bulb, which is surrounded by a socket called a hair follicle. The hair grows upwards from the root and arises from the skin surface. Each hair has a separate growth cycle.

- Anagen phase – where the hair grows in length
- Telogen phase – resting phase
- Catagen phase – where the hair is shed and falls out.

Different hairs all over the body will be at different stages of their growth cycles and are shed and replaced at different times. The length of the growth cycle varies between the different sites on the body and between individuals. On the chin, the hair cycle lasts 16 months, the number of hairs in the anagen phase is 20 per cent and the anagen phase lasts nine weeks. On the bikini line the hair cycle lasts 18 months, the number of hairs in the anagen phase is 30 per cent and lasts 22 weeks.

The skin is continually producing more hair follicles so, even if a method of hair removal that destroys them is used, after some months new hairs will begin to appear.

Hair Reduction and Removal

Permanent hair removal is the complete destruction of a hair follicle's ability to regenerate and grow new hair. If done correctly, electrolysis can achieve this. Permanent hair reduction refers to the stable reduction in the number of coarse dark hairs. This is achievable with laser and IPL treatment.

It must be appreciated that no method is 100 per cent effective in all clients. Some, for unknown reasons, do not respond at all to a given technique. Not all claims about the length of time for the hair to re-grow after treatment are necessarily accurate. 'Permanent' generally refers to being hair free for a year or more. 'Long term' usually refers to being hair free for six months. 'Semi-permanent' usually lasts only a few weeks.

Methods of Hair Removal

Intense pulsed light (IPL)

IPL is now becoming one of the commonest methods used for hair removal (see also pages 122–123). The hair follicles are damaged by the pulsed light energy and subsequently fail to produce new hairs.

The fair-skinned, dark-haired individual is the ideal candidate for treatment although more modern machines are being developed which can treat most skin types and hair colours.

A gel is applied to the skin. The gel has special properties so that the light energy is directed to the treatment area and reflections are avoided. Very intense light can damage the eyes and precautions have to be taken to ensure that reflections are kept to a minimum. A hand-held unit is then placed over the area covered by the gel and pulses of light are fired over the skin. This destroys the hair follicles and when the gel is removed, much of the hair is removed with it. The remaining hair in the treated areas usually falls out within two weeks.

Because of the number of different phases of the hair-growth cycle, about five or six treatments are necessary to obtain a favourable result. Results are not permanent, and further treatments will be required in the future.

Lasers

In recent years, lasers have come to the fore in removing unwanted hair. More lasers are being successfully developed to treat this problem. The light energy from the laser is absorbed by the pigment in the hair bulb and shaft. The duration of each laser pulse (a tiny fraction of a second) is accurately predetermined to heat and destroy the hair follicle but not to damage the surrounding skin and cause a burn. This process is called 'selective photothermolysis'.

The process is called 'selective' because it targets only the hair through its melanin pigment and not the skin (fair skin only). It must be appreciated that skin also contains melanin pigment so that the ideal candidate for hair removal has coarse dark hair against fair skin. Those with dark skin are not usually such good candidates for hair removal.

Hair that is coarser and more darkly pigmented responds best. Another important factor in terms of success is the percentage of unwanted hair that is actively growing. This varies from site to site e.g. up to 65 per cent actively growing hairs on the upper lip compared to only 20 per cent on the arms and legs.

Permanent laser hair removal is only effective on the actively growing (anagen phase) hairs. Several treatments will therefore be necessary in order to treat those hairs that were not at the correct phase of development during the previous treatment. Thus each area to be treated has to have a carefully compiled personalised treatment plan that not only considers the timing of successive treatment sessions but also adopts the optimum parameters necessary to ensure a successful result, e.g. pulse duration (length of time a laser pulse is passed), fluence (quantity of energy delivered to the skin) and delay (length of time between two pulses).

To reduce pain and discomfort during the procedure, a spray of cool gas or air is used to allow the skin to be properly cooled when the laser beam hits it.

Postoperative events

Pain   Usually pain is not severe and much less than after electrolysis, so local anaesthetic is usually not necessary. Those with a low pain threshold or who find the procedure unpleasant can apply local anaesthetic cream before treatment. Oral sedatives can be prescribed for the very nervous patient prior to treatment.

Redness   Redness of the skin and slight crusting may occur and after two or three days the skin may become flaky. Using a moisturiser will help to minimise this effect.

Pigmentation   Pigmentation changes of the skin can occur afterwards especially in patients with dark coloured skin where lightening of the skin can be seen. In those who tan easily, darkening of the skin can be seen (post-inflammatory pigmentation) and may take several months to fade. In all such cases a skin test should be performed first to determine suitability for treatment.

   Women who have had melasma (pigmentation change on the face usually associated with pregnancy or taking the contraceptive pill) have a high risk of suffering from colour changes. Treatment is therefore contraindicated.

Long-term sequelae   There does not appear to be a long-term risk of skin disorders or skin cancer.

Latest technology

As mentioned previously, laser technology is constantly being improved. The latest device combines laser energy with bi-polar radio-frequency energy to attain superior results using lower energy output. This means a higher level of safety and far less discomfort for the patient. In addition it removes hair of all colours on all skin types. Long-term results are still being evaluated.

   If you are seeking hair-removal treatment you are best advised to research your local providers carefully in order to ensure you receive the best treatment possible.

Electrolysis

Electrolysis refers to the destruction of hair roots with an electric current. It was, until recently, by far the most common and effective technique for permanent hair removal. It is still very widely available. This method is now declining in popularity as more advanced technology, such as lasers, has become available. The methods of electrolysis available are:

1. Galvanic – A direct current (DC) passing through a needle causes a chemical reaction in the hair follicle, which produces sodium hydroxide and destroys the hair follicle. This method is most often used to remove the upper lip and chin hairs.

2. Thermolysis – An alternating current (AC) passing through a needle causes vibration in the water molecules surrounding the hair follicle. The heat generated damages the hair follicle. This is also known as 'short-wave radio-frequency diathermy'.

3. The blend method combines the two above.

Method

With the aid of a strong magnifying glass, a very fine metal needle is inserted into the hair follicle and an electric current is passed along it, which destroys the hair root. Each hair has to be treated individually and the technique is therefore time consuming and takes several sessions. Many women opt for a two-sessions-per-month plan until all the hairs have been treated. In successful cases, it may be several years before significant regrowth occurs. The hairs to be treated have to be well developed and visible before treatment, so you have to go through a stage of having significant amounts of unwanted hair before you can get them removed. If you have very curly hair, the hair follicles won't be straight and it is difficult to get the needle to go all along the follicle right to its end. This reduces the effectiveness of the electric current and, although it weakens the hair growth, further sessions on the same follicle may be required to completely eradicate it. Electrolysis works for all hair colours.

Side effects

These include discomfort and pain, redness, swelling, dryness and scabbing. In untrained hands, or in those patients who tend to scar badly, permanent pitted scarring can result due to surrounding skin damage. The numerous tiny pits that can occur with each session of electrolysis can eventually build up to produce an uneven scarred area and thickened, coarse skin. This scarring is however amenable to treatment by dermabrasion (see pages 110–113) or laser skin resurfacing (see pages 119–122). It is a tedious and lengthy technique compared to laser and IPL treatment (see above).

Results

Electrolysis is often viewed as a permanent method because once destroyed, the hair will not grow back. Several sessions are necessary to ensure a successful result.

Nowadays, with the advent of more refined technology, electrolysis is perhaps best suited to situations where there are less than a dozen hairs to remove. This treatment is more likely to be offered in beauty salons than in the cosmetic surgeon's office. It has the added advantage that it is suitable for all hair colours and treatment is less expensive than other treatments.

Sound Waves

New technology has harnessed the use of ultrasonic (very high frequency) sound waves, which can numb the follicle (to minimise discomfort) and then pass through the hair in a fraction of a second. This results in disintegration of the hair-follicle cells without damaging the surrounding tissue. The hair is painlessly removed.

Method

The area to be treated is cleansed and a lotion massaged into the area. Each hair is gripped by tweezers and simultaneously thousands of ultrasonic sound waves are passed through the hair in a fraction of a second. As sound takes the path of least resistance it travels down the porous hair shaft to strike and disintegrate the hair follicle. The hair is then easily and gently pulled out with the tweezers.

Results

The time interval between treatments is usually recommended to be two to three weeks. Although all the hairs are quickly removed in one session there will be some regrowth, especially when the hair is not in the anagen stage (see above).

Side effects are minimal and all areas of the body can be safely treated. The advantages of this system are that:

- It is non-invasive
- It is pain free
- there is no risk of burning the skin because no heat is generated
- there is therefore no risk of scarring or pitting
- it is safe for diabetics.

Make-up can be applied 10 minutes after treatment. The safety of this treatment means it is readily available in beauty salons and is rapidly becoming one of the most popular hair-removal systems available.

Summary

It is difficult to recommend which of the above hair-removal treatments is best because each one has its advantages and disadvantages. In addition, every situation is unique and patient preference will no doubt influence the final decision. Operator preference and recommendation will also play a large part in the final decision.

The table on the following page shows the relevant points, which should be considered when selecting the technique best suited for each situation.

Electrolysis	Laser/IPL	Sound waves
Uses electric current, which generates heat or initiates chemical reaction	Uses light energy	Use static and sound waves
Risk of scabbing or permanently scarring the skin	Risk of burning, pigmentation and de-pigmentation and possibly scarring	Non-invasive, no risk of damaging the skin
Very painful	Uncomfortable	Almost painless
Thins an area of hair. Adjacent hair cannot be treated	Complete clearance in one session	Complete clearance of area in one session
Removal from sensitive areas can be painful	Some areas cannot be treated e.g. eyebrows	All areas can be treated
No make-up for 24 hours	No make-up for 24 hours	Make-up after 30 minutes
Not advised on sensitive skin	Not advised on sensitive skin	Can be used on all skin types
Can be used on all hair and skin types	Only suitable for pale skin with dark hair	Can use on all hair and skin types

Correction of Muscle and Bony Defects

CALF AUGMENTATION

There are two groups of people who seek this operation. The first consists of those who have had an injury or a disease, such as polio or clubfoot, which has affected muscle development in one or both legs. The other group consists of those who have normal legs but the calf region is proportionately too thin, causing embarrassment. In both groups the treatment is essentially the same, which is to insert a soft silicone calf implant to plump out the affected part.

The operation

Under a general anaesthetic, with you lying on your front, the surgeon will make an incision in the natural crease line at the back of the knee. A pocket for the implant is made over the affected muscle and the correctly sized and shaped implant is inserted.

The procedure can be performed on a day-care basis although an overnight stay in the clinic is perhaps best advised. Walking is encouraged immediately afterwards.

Postoperative events

Bruising and swelling Bruising and swelling of the foot can occur and usually resolves in a few days.

Infection Infection is uncommon, but if it occurs it can occasionally necessitate the temporary removal of the implant while the infection subsides. A second procedure at a later date will be necessary to reinsert the implant.

Scars These are usually about 5cm (2in) long and lie in the natural crease at the back of the knee. They usually heal satisfactorily.

Encapsulation Encapsulation can occur as with breast implants (see pages 148–149) but this is uncommon. The body will form a layer of scar tissue around the implant after about 10 days. This scar tissue may thicken, contract or do both after a period of time. It may be associated with discomfort, which in some cases will necessitate the removal of the implant and enlarging the pocket further.

Asymmetry Asymmetry is more common after surgery if there is a marked asymmetry preoperatively. Perfect symmetry is simply not possible in many cases.

Sensory changes Sensations such as shooting pains and temporary loss of feeling can often occur. Sensation usually returns fully to normal after a few weeks.

Rupture of implant This may rarely occur spontaneously, but is mostly associated with trauma, such as the calf being struck heavily.

Deep vein thrombosis (DVT) DVT is the most serious complication that can occur postoperatively, but thankfully it is rare. Stopping smoking, early postoperative walking, and cessation of oral contraceptives are perhaps the best preventative measures in helping to avoid this complication.

Implant displacement On rare occasions the implant can be displaced (usually as a direct result of trauma) and lie in an unusual position. Further surgery will be necessary to correct this problem.

Results
When successfully performed, this procedure undoubtedly boosts self-confidence. It is however not a very popular operation and in some patients the results are not very realistic, especially if there wasn't very much muscle in the calf to start with. Usually the implant doesn't move in the same way that a muscle would on walking.

SUNKEN CHEST OR PECTUS EXCAVATUM

This inherited condition, where the central wall of the chest is sunken or depressed in varying degrees of severity, predominantly affects males. Occasionally the deformity is so severe that it affects breathing and requires surgery to the bones of the rib cage to alter its shape. Less severe cases that have no functional breathing problems are adequately dealt with by inserting a suitably moulded silicone implant into the defect under the skin.

The operation

Before the operation, a mould is made of the depression in the chest. Using this mould, a silicone implant is specially manufactured in order to fill in the chest defect accurately. A trial fitting of the implant is done before the operation in the consulting room to ensure that it fits.

Under general anaesthetic an incision is made near the top of the depression and the implant is inserted into a pocket made between the skin and the front of the chest wall. Usually a drain is inserted to prevent fluid collection for the first 24 hours. You will usually be discharged home the following day.

Postoperative events

Scars A fine scar usually results, but as with all incisions on the front of the chest it may take many weeks to settle. The chest is an area of the body where scars can sometimes heal unfavourably and require further treatment e.g. steroid injections (see 'Improving Unsightly Scars, pages 196–199).

Pain and discomfort Strong painkillers will be necessary in the immediate postoperative period but standard ones usually suffice after a few days.

Collection of fluid Fluid collecting around the implant is quite common after surgery and will need to be drawn off (aspirated) with a needle. This is easily performed as an outpatient procedure. Several aspirations may be necessary before healing finally occurs.

Visible implant If the implant is not an exact fit, or if it moves slightly, the edges may become visible and this may require surgical correction.

Postoperative management
Patients are strongly advised to wear a support garment for the first three weeks to immobilise the implant thereby encouraging healing and reduce fluid collection. Sutures are removed after a week.

Results
The specially made implant is usually very effective at improving the contour of the skin and provides a very pleasing cosmetic result.

OTHER BONY DEFECTS

In parts of the body where bones lie close to the skin such as the shin bone, nose, jaw and skull etc., an irregularity or shallow dent can be treated by one of the many semi-permanent fillers that are available (see pages 102–106).

BUTTOCK CONTOURING

Buttock implants have become more popular recently as a result of media publicity highlighting the desirable buttock shapes of certain celebrities. Genetics and race play a major role in buttock shape and it is difficult if not impossible to change the underlying shape of buttocks through exercise. Few surgeons currently perform buttock implantation in the UK, primarily because it is not an easy procedure and because in inexperienced hands the incidence of failure is high.

The buttock area is subjected to many stresses and movements during walking and sitting, therefore it is vitally important to ensure that the operation is expertly and accurately performed in order to reduce the incidence of postoperative complications.

There are two options currently available: inserting a custom-made silicone buttock implant behind the main buttock muscle, or transferring unwanted fat (usually from the abdomen) to the buttock.

Buttock Implants
The operation
You will be admitted on the day of the operation, which is usually performed under general anaesthesia. Lying on your front, the surgeon will make a 6–8cm (2½–3in) vertical midline incision in the crease (crack)

between the buttocks. Through this incision a suitable pocket is made within or beneath the buttock muscle. Some surgeons make a pocket under the fibrous lining of the buttock muscle. A specially designed silicone buttock implant is inserted into the pocket. Both sides can be augmented through the one midline incision. Buttock implants are solid shapes made of soft silicone and are available in various shapes and sizes.

Implant size and shape is largely determined at preoperative consultation after a detailed discussion and the agreement of both you and your surgeon. The final decision is made at the operation. Fine adjustments can be made by carving the implant in order to obtain the best fit.

After the operation the incision is sutured and a taped pressure dressing is applied in order to reduce postoperative discomfort and swelling. When the dressing is removed a few days later an elastic compression garment is fitted and worn for three weeks.

Postoperative events

Pain and discomfort You will usually experience more pain and discomfort than with most other cosmetic procedures and recovery is usually longer. After five to seven days, walking and sitting down will become more tolerable. Some surgeons advise not to sit for a few days after the operation. The taped dressing is usually removed after two to three days when a shower may be taken.

Infection It must be appreciated that this area is particularly liable to become infected. Extra precautions are taken during surgery and you must follow postoperative directions meticulously to try to avoid this complication. The more experienced surgeon who regularly performs this procedure will have fewer infections in his patients than the inexperienced.

Bleeding and haematoma The surgeon must take every precaution to minimise the risk of postoperative bleeding with the possible development of a haematoma, which would necessitate a further procedure to drain it.

Slippage The implant can move and cause an abnormal shape and asymmetry of the buttocks. Due to the stress placed on the buttocks during sitting, walking and running, any implant situated in this region will suffer intense forces from movement. An implant can thus easily be moved out of position.

Asymmetry   Perfect symmetry is the aim, rarely the achievement. Some asymmetry will occur no matter how well the operation has been performed. Gross asymmetry will have to be corrected with further surgery but minor degrees must be accepted. This is much less likely in experienced hands, as accurate placement is vital to the long-term result.

Recovery   Full activity may be resumed four weeks after surgery. It is important to realise that it will take several weeks for the tissues to stretch adequately to give the final shape. It can take as long as six to eight months before the implants feel like part of your body and no longer feel strange.

Fat Transfer

Some surgeons claim they get consistently good results by using the technique of fat transfer. In this procedure fat is harvested from another part of the body, usually the abdomen, and transferred to the buttock region to give it more volume and shape. Unfortunately many patients seeking buttock enlargement are thin and have very little donor fat available. In those that have an abundance of fat, reducing the donor area will also help to create a more pleasing contour in that area.

The operation

The procedure is usually carried out as a day case. Fat is harvested under local or general anaesthetic (usually from the abdominal wall), washed, prepared and injected into the recipient area of the buttocks. The redundant fat is stored for subsequent top-up injections because some of the injected fat will be absorbed. Repeat injections can be performed at six-week intervals.

Postoperative events

Postoperatively it is recommended not to sit for at least five days in order to create the optimum conditions for the fat to 'take'. Mild to moderate pain, discomfort and swelling should be expected. Other complications are as for liposuction in general (see pages 168–173). The size of buttock enlargement that is possible with a fat implant is really quite limited and it takes repeated injections to achieve a visible difference.

Conclusion –
The Future of
Cosmetic Surgery

The science of surgery has a huge respect for tradition and also a very healthy interest in the new and the bold. If we look back at what surgeons were doing 200 years ago, from our perspective many of their techniques would seem crude and brutal. It makes one wonder what the surgeons in 200 years time will think of us! At the present time the rate of development of medical science and technology has never been greater. All over the world surgeons are bubbling with ideas and keen to try them out.

And yet, quite a few of the operations performed regularly today are still more or less the same, even in a rapidly moving field like cosmetic surgery, as they were 150 years ago. The limiting and constant factor is the human body, which has stayed the same for centuries.

Many surgeons accept that it is the advances that have been made in anaesthetics that have really pushed the boundaries outwards and made modern surgery possible. To undergo an operation in relative comfort and with only a tiny risk involved would have been only a dream a few decades ago.

Anaesthetics are now safe, in the sense that you are taking a greater risk every time you get into a car. Recovery from anaesthesia is now speedier and far less unpleasant than it was previously. Modern drugs to combat postoperative nausea and vomiting have drastically reduced unpleasant side effects.

Whereas a generation or two ago, people may only have considered surgery for life and death situations, women are now perfectly prepared to undergo major surgery for what would have been considered trivial reasons years ago. Advances in surgical techniques mean that one no longer has to put up with a deformity or imperfection; you can get it fixed.

This change in philosophy and the improvement in the safety, comfort and effectiveness of modern surgery have hugely increased the number of people willing to undergo cosmetic surgery.

There is also far greater peer pressure exerted in our communities to look our best. People are slimming, exercising and giving up smoking all over the world. Many developed countries have an obesity problem that is of huge concern to the medical health authorities. Conversely, there are far more 'beautiful people' around, on our TV screens and in the media.

The huge growth in the worldwide demand for cosmetic surgery in recent years has undoubtedly led to many new developments and ideas. Many have initially taken off, only to be thwarted once the long-term adverse effects become apparent. A few have taken the world of cosmetic surgery by storm, most notably Botox®, which is now probably the most popular, minimally invasive cosmetic treatment in the world. To date, the long-term adverse effects of Botox® have either not occurred or have not come to the fore. We suspect that sooner or later a long-term side effect will become established. Only time will tell.

We believe that the standard, established surgical procedures will continue to be popular in the immediate future and will not undergo dramatic changes, apart from, perhaps, specific minor refinements which are usually a matter of personal choice for each individual surgeon. Most surgeons will eventually adopt a technique with specific personal refinements that work for them, based on past experience and patient satisfaction. It is seldom seen for two surgeons to perform a complex surgical procedure in exactly the same manner. Even using different suture materials is a major difference.

The majority of changes will occur with the advent of new technology, which will either be a new, sole procedure or combined with a standard surgical procedure. An example of this is the combination of liposuction with face lifting or abdominoplasty.

The goal of any new development is to produce a technique or treatment that is quick, painless, has the minimum recovery time, and is relatively inexpensive. In addition it must be relatively easy for the surgeon to learn and master, or complications and adverse sequelae will be common. Liposuction is a relatively easy procedure to learn, but the number of serious complications and unacceptably poor results over the years has been high. The so-called 'lunchtime' treatment is the ultimate aim as this enhances the popularity of any procedure.

The current demands of most cosmetic surgeons, in order of importance, would be to be able to perform operations without producing scars, to control and enhance the healing process and to be able to treat certain conditions that were previously difficult if impossible to treat e.g. stretch marks on the body. Although much research and development has been done in this field already, results are far from ideal to date.

New Devices

Lasers

Lasers have undoubtedly revolutionised medicine in recent years and new ones are constantly being introduced that claim to be superior to previous models. In the field of cosmetic surgery newer and more successful developments for hair and tattoo removal will undoubtedly come to the fore in the not-too-distant future.

Newer lasers are being developed for skin resurfacing that will give more successful results without the drawn-out healing process and recovery time associated with the current generation of lasers, which have precluded many patients from undergoing treatment.

There is increasing awareness of the skin-damaging effect of sunlight. Hopefully women who are young now will have much better facial skin than their mothers, who were brought up to believe that a dark tan was healthy. Research has shown that it certainly is not.

Radiofrequency devices

Radiofrequency devices are being used increasingly for facial rejuvenation and we feel that this area has much to offer in the future. It is currently of benefit for mild aging but will not tighten up the loose tissues associated with the usual patient who seeks facial rejuvenation surgery.

Perhaps a combination of a laser and radiofrequency device, or even a completely new technology hitherto untried, will offer more exciting prospects in the future.

Facial fillers

Newer, safer and longer lasting fillers are constantly being developed and this will undoubtedly continue with a kinder method of administration in the form of painless injections. Tissue-culture technology was in use for the last few years in Britain, although it was very expensive. There have been some successful results, but unfortunately this treatment has recently been withdrawn due to closure of the company. It is likely to be restarted at some point, hopefully with less expense for the patient.

Current Surgical Procedures

There is little doubt that many of the procedures popular today will become obsolete in the future as newer techniques and developments come to the fore. Invisible scars will one day become a reality, so perhaps a revolutionary surgical speciality will emerge.

Newer and less invasive techniques for fat reduction will be developed, making the traditional liposuction procedure obsolete. Perhaps a combination of oral preparations and safer injections for selective fat reduction will become available in the not too distant future.

In the field of breast surgery, a safe, oral preparation for augmentation without the need of implants will one day be a reality. Breast reduction and uplift will take the form of shrinkage of breast tissue with oral preparations as well as non- or minimally invasive techniques for skin tightening utilising a device that will shrink skin.

Less invasive treatments for the loose abdomen following pregnancy will offer tightening procedures for skin and muscle as well as eliminate stretch marks and cellulite.

Surgically invasive procedures for facial rejuvenation will cease and minimally or non-invasive 'lunchtime' procedures will become the norm.

There have recently been a few, very well publicised face transplants. Unfortunately, the problem with such surgery is not the difficulty or complexity of the surgery. The real problem is that the skin is part of the body's defence system against infection and it reacts very strongly in the presence of any foreign material. Skin used as a graft is likely to fight the host, while the host tries to reject the skin. This is why living skin grafts can only be taken from the patient's own body. Killed, sterilised skin from someone else is a very poor substitute. A patient having a face transplant will face a lifetime of strong immunosuppressive drugs. In the long term, this will increase the risk of cancer (because the immune system holds cancer in check) and a succession of serious life-threatening infections. Most surgeons feel it is too soon to undertake face transplant surgery until these rejection problems are solved. However, the pioneers of this treatment say that their patients are so disfigured that they have no life at all, so giving them a short life with some semblance of normality is a huge benefit.

Genetic Engineering

This is, without doubt, the ultimate or 'mother' of all treatments, but still a fantasy and a very long way away. If man ever becomes adept at being able to alter the genetic structure of a human being in a controlled and efficient manner it will completely revolutionise our world. Apart from being able to successfully treat, or even eradicate, incurable diseases it would be possible to control the aging process, change skin colour, choose our body shape etc. – the list goes on.

It should not be too long before it is possible to grow complete organs by taking a few cells from a patient and culturing them in a laboratory. The cosmetic industry will certainly get in on this and, in a generation or two, or maybe even sooner, it will be possible to 'grow' a brand new face and seamlessly attach it, having removed the old one. This will solve the rejection problems associated with trying to graft someone else's skin.

Infection

When antibiotics were first used it was thought that eventually we would be able to abolish all pathological infections. Unfortunately, bacteria evolve at a stupendous rate and have always managed to keep one step ahead of any medical steps we may take to counter them. Indeed, infection with bacteria that are resistant to nearly all antibiotics is a serious problem in many of our hospitals. It would be a huge advance if we could operate without any risk of infection.

The Control of Scarring

One of the limitations of current cosmetic surgery is that nearly all operations produce scars, this being the way that the body repairs itself after injury. It was noticed some time ago that injuries to unborn babies rarely, if ever, produce scars. This means that there must be a way for the body to repair itself without scar formation, if only we could find it and control the process. We know a lot about how the healing process is initiated after an injury; there is a series of very complex chemicals released into the injured area, which is in some analogous to the blood clotting mechanism – another highly complex biochemical process. These chemicals produced after injury cause new cells to migrate into the area, open up blood vessels (so the healing area swells) and make many types of cells grow and multiply, which they wouldn't normally do.

The end result of all this activity is to produce a mesh of fibrous tissue that closes the wound securely, preventing further injury and infection. This is the scar. Although a lot is known about how the process starts, very little is known about what stops it once healing is complete. In some patients, this mechanism is defective and scars continue to grow unabated until they are much bigger than the original wound. This is commonly seen in persons of black African descent.

So, the really big advance we are all waiting for is a method of controlling wound healing so that scars never form and the skin shows no sign of any injury. That advance will certainly be on a par with the development of safe anaesthesia and the invention of antibiotics.

It would also be desirable, when we understand more about the intricate mechanism of healing and the response to injury, to minimise the bruising and swelling phase, which is such a problem with present day surgery.

On the Starship Enterprise, Dr Leonard 'Bones' McCoy is able to cure patients with life-threatening conditions just by waving a gadget near them. Should this ever become a reality many people currently working in the cosmetic industry, including your authors, will become unemployed. We will then look back at our long careers and maybe just say, 'Wow!'

After many years as practising surgeons in this most rewarding of specialities we can reminisce and be grateful that we were practising at a time when cosmetic surgery finally became acceptable, and that we were able to witness the huge growth and development of our chosen field.

A Final Note

We sincerely hope you enjoyed reading this book and gained the information you were seeking in order to give you an initial realistic insight into what is involved when considering undergoing a cosmetic surgical procedure. It goes without saying that to gain full insight, a consultation with the operating surgeon (and no other party) is essential in order to be in a position to make an informed decision about proceeding with surgery.

In our experience, most women contemplating cosmetic surgery are seeking to improve a particular aspect of their external anatomy and simply wish to appear 'normal'. It is therefore important not to be swept along on a tide of media sensationalism of either extreme, whether it be the disaster stories or the idea that it can be done in a lunch hour with no side effects whatsoever.

It is extremely important to feel comfortable with your chosen surgeon, so an important step is to do your homework and select one that you feel you can trust. Of course it is not always that easy and you may need to have more than one consultation with a particular surgeon, as well as others with different surgeons, in order to decide which is the one for you.

Many patients have said that the freedom to wear the clothes and hairstyle they always wanted without feeling self-conscious has given them an enormous boost and has allowed them to live the life they always dreamt of. However, if the result of cosmetic surgery is disappointing – and it occasionally is – then it can be an experience to bitterly regret.

In some cases a revision procedure will be necessary. There are many reasons for this. It may not necessarily be simply because of incompetent or inadequate surgery, because surgery is not an exact science and results can never be promised or guaranteed. Whereas there are poorly skilled or reckless practitioners in this field, irreversible disasters are extremely rare.

Cosmetic surgery is not for everyone. If performed by a competent surgeon in a patient who is self motivated; has an obvious blemish which is eminently correctable by surgery; understands the procedure as well as the likely limitations, postoperative sequelae and complications; as well as has realistic expectations, results are excellent in the vast majority of cases and patients need not be apprehensive and should proceed with confidence. If however these criteria are not met, the result can be disappointing and the patient and surgeon will live to regret proceeding in the first place.

Finally, you should always consider that a successful outcome from a cosmetic surgery procedure can be very rewarding and even life changing, as it will give you increased confidence and self-esteem.

APPENDIX
GLOSSARY

Advertorial	Text in a newspaper or magazine that purports to be editorial but is really an advertisement, often paid for by the subject of the article.
Alopecia	Medical term for baldness. From the Greek for 'fox mange'.
Anticoagulant	An agent that reduces the ability of the blood to clot. Some drugs, e.g. aspirin have this effect and can considerably increase bruising after operations or injury or even cause severe bleeding. Anticoagulants are used therapeutically in the treatment of thrombosis, see 'coagulant' below.
Antiplatelet	Platelets are tiny cells in the blood that play an essential role in blood clotting. An antiplatelet agent reduces their function and can initiate bruising or bleeding.
Cannula	Tube that can be inserted into the body to inject or withdraw fluid. Liposuction cannulae are usually made of metal. The word is derived from the Latin word meaning 'a small cane'. Hollow canes were used historically before modern technology enabled the use of metal or plastic.
Coagulant	An agent that helps the blood to clot. It is essential that the blood can clot, so that blood loss is reduced after injury. Clot formation is a very complex process and many substances affect the process. If a blood clot occurs inappropriately in a blood vessel, without being caused by an injury, it is called a thrombosis. The clot may travel in the bloodstream and form a blockage in another vessel, causing serious or even fatal consequences.
Coumarin	Chemical found in many plants. It has an anticoagulant effect in animals.
Complications	Events following a treatment that are not part of the normal healing process.
Cosmetic surgery	Surgery that aims to change the appearance for the better in the absence of any pathology. It is also known as aesthetic (or beautifying) surgery. If there is an obvious pathology such as a burn or scar then the surgery is spoken of as being plastic or reconstructive.

Dermis	The deep layer of the skin. It is mainly made of collagen with a few elastic fibres. It is the main constituent of leather. It also contains the glands and hair follicles.
Dorsum	Latin for back. As part of the nose it means the bony ridge at the front of the nose running from the forehead to the tip.
—ectomy	An operation to cut something out. From the Greek word for 'excision'.
Elective	Of an operation, it means at the option of the doctor or patient, and implies that it is not urgently or medically necessary.
Epidermis	The outside layer of the skin. It is made up of several layers of cells. New cells are being continuously produced in the deeper layers and they gradually get flatter as they near the surface and are eventually shed.
Glabella	The area between the eyebrows.
Invasive treatment	Treatment, such as surgery, in which the body's surface is cut or opened to allow access beneath the skin.
Maxillofacial	Description of a branch of surgery that specialises in treating the face, especially the mouth and jaws. Maxillofacial surgeons are usually qualified dentists as well as medical doctors.
Necrosis	The death or decay of (or part of) an organ or tissue as a result of disease or lack of nutrients. If skin necrosis occurs after surgery it can be due to lack of blood supply or infection. This can occur if the skin is stretched too tight, or if swelling beneath the skin, such as from a haematoma, impedes the blood supply. Smoking damages the tiny blood vessels in the skin and heavy smokers are more vulnerable to this complication. If the area is large, it would cause devastating scarring.
—oma	A swelling or lump. The cause is the first part of the word, so a swelling due to a collection of blood is a 'haema-toma'.
Oral commissure	The fleshy lump felt and seen just lateral to the mouth opening on each side. It is where the muscle fibres of the upper lip intermesh with those of the lower lip. These muscles tend to be well developed in wind instrument players. Patients sometimes notice these lumps and complain about them often after facelifting.
—otomy	An operation that cuts into something. From the Greek word 'to cut'.

Pathological	Involving or caused by the nature of disease or illness.
—pexy	An operation to place something in a better position. From the Greek word meaning 'to fix or put together'.
—plasty	An operation to change the shape. From the Latin word that means 'to mould'. A plastic is a substance that can be moulded, such as when it is heated.
Revision	A second or subsequent operation or procedure that aims to improve the result of the first.
Rosacea	Medical condition in which the blood vessels in the skin enlarge, producing a flushed look. Often the skin thickens in chronic cases. Tends to be seen over the cheeks and on the nose and is exacerbated by sun exposure.
Salicylate	Chemical found in several plants that is related to aspirin, and therefore has an anticoagulant effect.
Sequelae	A disease or condition occurring as the result of a previous disease or accident. Usually in plural. Can also mean simply 'that which follows'. Directly from the Latin.
Subdermal	Just underneath the skin. Subcuticular means the same.
Unfavourable	Literally it means 'not looked upon with favour', but in medical usage it means a disappointing or poor result.
Viable	Likely or able to survive or live. In medical usage, if a part of the body such as an area of skin is deprived of its blood supply it may not be viable in which case it will die. The resulting skin defect will cause a bad scar. Viability means having the attribute of being viable.
Vital signs	Specific features of a body that are associated with life. In medical terminology it means the pulse rate, the blood pressure, the oxygen level in the blood and the breathing rate. All of these are monitored continuously during a general anaesthetic.

APPENDIX
COMMON DIETARY HERBS THAT MIGHT AFFECT SURGERY

Agrimony
(Agrimonia eupatoria, agromonia, cockle-bur): Coagulant effect from vitamin K constituent.

Alfalfa
(Medicago sativa, lucerne, purple medick): Anticoagulant effect from coumarin constituents and coagulant effect from vitamin K.

Angelica
(Angelica archangelica, root of the Holy Ghost): Anticoagulant and antiplatelet effect from coumarin constituents.

Anise
(Pimpinella anisum, aniseed, sweet cumin): Anticoagulant effect from excessive doses from coumarin constituents.

Arnica
(Arnica montana, leopard's bane, wolf's bane, mountain tobacco): Anticoagulant effect from coumarin constituents.

Asafoetida
(Ferula assa-foetida, assant, fum, giant fennel, devil's dung): Anticoagulant from coumarin constituents.

Aspen
(Populi cortex, Populi folium): Antiplatelet effect from salicin constituent.

Black cohosh
(Cimicifuga racemosa, bugwort snakeroot, baneberry): Antiplatelet effect from salicylate constituent.

Bogbean
(Menyanthes trifoliata, water shamrock, buck-bean, marsh trefoil): Bleeding risk from unknown constituent.

Boldo
(Peumus boldus, boldine): Anticoagulant effect from coumarin constituents.

Borage Seed Oil
(Borago officinalis, starflower, burage): Anticoagulant effect from gamma linolenic acid and antiplatelet effect.

Bromelain
(Ananas comosus, bromelin): Anticoagulant effect from enzyme constituent.

Capsicum
(Capsicum frutescen, African pepper, cayenne, chili pepper): Antiplatelet effect from capsaicinoid constituents.

Celery
(Apium graveolens, smallage, Apii fructus): Antiplatelet effect from apiogenin (coumarin) constituent.

Clove
(Syzygium aromaticum, caryophyllus) Antiplatelet effect from eugenol constituent.

Danshen
(Salvia miltiorrhiza, red sage, salvia root): Anticoagulant effect from protocatechualdehyde 3,4-dihydroxyphenyl-lactic acid constituent.

Dong Quai	(Angelica sinensis, Danggui, Chinese angelica): Anticoagulant and antiplatelet from coumarin constituents.
European Mistletoe	(Viscum album, devil's fuge, dru-denfuss, all-heal): Coagulant effect from lectin constituent.
Fenugreek	(Trigonella foenum-graecum, bird's foot, Greek hay): Anticoagulant effect from coumarin constituents.
Feverfew	(Tanacetum parthenium, bachelor's button, featherfew, midsummer daisy): Antiplatelet effect from the crude extracts.
Fish Oils	(omega-3 fatty acids): Antiplatelet effect with prostacyclin synthesis, vasodilatation, reduced platelets and adhesiveness, and prolonged bleeding time.
Fucus	(Fucus vesiculosis, kelp, black tang, bladder wrack, cutweed): Anticoagulant effect which can increase the risk of bleeding.
Garlic	(Allium sativum, nectar of the gods, stinking rose): Inhibition of platelet aggregation and can increase risk of bleeding in excessive doses.
Ginger	(Zingiber officinale): Anticoagulant effect with increased risk of bleeding.
Ginkgo	(Ginkgo biloba, maidenhair): Inhibits platelet aggregation and decreases blood viscosity
Ginseng	(Panax ginseng, Asian ginseng, Korean red, jintsam): Anticoagulant and antiplatelet effects.
Goldenseal	(Hydrastis canadensis, eye balm, yellow puccoon): Coagulant effect from berberine constituent.
Horse Chestnut	(Aesculus hippocastanum, escine, venostat): Anticoagulant effect from aesculin (coumarin) constituent.
Horseradish	(Armoracia rusticana, pepperrot, mountain radish): Anticoagulant effect from coumarin constituents.
Liquorice	(Glycyrrhiza glabra, sweet root): Antiplatelet effect from coumarin constituent.
Meadowseet	(Filipendula ulmania, bridewort, dropwort): Anticoagulant effect from salicylate constituents.
Northern Prickly Ash	(Xanthoxylum americanum, pepper wood, toothache bark): Anticoagulant effect from coumarin constituents.
Onion	(Allium cepa): Antiplatelet effect from unknown constituent.
Papain	(Carica papaya): Bleeding risk from unknown constituent.
Passionflower	(Passiflora incarnata, apricot vine, Maypop): Anticoagulant effect from coumarin constituents.
Pau D'Arco	(Tabebuia ampetiginosa, ipes, taheebo tea, lapacho): Anticoagulant effect from lapachol constituent.
Plantain	(Plantago major, common plantain, greater plantain): Coagulant effect from vitamin K constituent.
Poplar	(Populus tacamahacca, balm of Gilead) Antiplatelet effect from salicin constituent.

Quassia (Quassia amara, bittenwood): Anticoagulant effect from coumarin constituents.

Red Clover (Trifolium praetense, trefoil, cow clover, beebread): Anticoagulant effect from coumarin constituents.

Roman Chamomile (Chamaemelum nobile, English chamomile, whig plant, garden chamomile) Anticoagulant effect from coumarin constituents.

Safflower (Carthamus tinctorium, saffron, zaffer) Anticoagulant effect from safflower yellow constituent.

Southern Prickly Ash (Zanthoxylum clava-herculis, sea ash, yellow wood): Anticoagulant effect from coumarin constituents.

Stinging Nettle (Urtica diolca, nettle): Coagulant effect from vitamin K constituent.

Sweet Clover (Melilotus officinalis, hay flower, common melilot, sweet lucerne): Anticoagulant effect from dicumarol constituent.

Sweet Vernal Grass (Anthoxanthum odoratum, spring grass): Anticoagulant effect from coumarin constituent.

Tonka Bean (Dipterux odorata, coumarouna, torquin bean): Anticoagulant effect from coumarin constituent.

Vitamin E (Alpha-tocopherol): Inhibits platelet aggregation and adhesion and interferes with vitamin-K dependent clotting factor in large doses.

INDEX

folding 150
leakage 152
lifespan 153
operation 146–7
problems 53
protrusion 150–1
reasons for having 143
rejection of 153
removal 154
safety 155–7
shape 144
structural variations 144–5
surface 144
types 143–4
wrinkling 150
breast reduction 20, 161–5
operation 162–3
postoperative events 163–4
postoperative management 164
preoperative consultation 161–2
breast uplift 157–61, 162
operation 159
postoperative events 159
postoperative management 160
preoperative consultation 158–9
breasts:
cancer of 154
drooping 150, 157
investigations 149–50
lumps in 150
nipples:
inversion 164
correction 165–7
loss of 165
sensitivity 151–2
surgery 142–67, 223
British Association of Cosmetic
Surgeons (BACS) 24–7, 34
Code of Practice 25–7
contacting 32
brow lift 85–7
endoscopic 86–7
postoperative events 86, 87
traditional 85–6

bruising 39
bullying 17
buttock contouring 217–19

C
cadaver implants 92, 93
calf augmentation 214–15
Capacitive Radiofrequency (CRF)
124–5
capsular contracture 148–9
cellulite 223
cellulitis 39
cheeks 88–91
implants 88–90
autologous fat 90
postoperative events 89
synthetic injectable 91
cheiloplasty 91–2
chemical peeling chemabrasion 101,
109–10, 113–15
postoperative events 114–15
chest, sunken 216–17
chest infections 40, 49, 63
childhood 17
chin:
augmentation 138–41
operation 138–9
postoperative events 139
double-chin removal 87–8
receding 140
circulation, impaired 49
clinic, routine admission to 64–7
clitoral reduction 182–3
clotting disorders 48
Code of Practice 24–7
cold sores 110
collagen 102–3
complications 30, 36–41, 59
see also individual procedure
from surgery abroad 35
conjunctival chemosis 98
consultants 21–2

fillers:
    for chin 140–1
    facial 222
    fat transfer 106–7, 219
    implants 108
    permanent 107–8
    temporary 100, 101–6
flap necrosis 49, 78, 81, 83, 178
food, abstinence from 50
freckles 119

G
G-spot implant 182
general practitioners, referral by 32–3
genetic engineering 223–4
genital cosmetic surgery 180–3
glossary 228–30
glycolic acid 113

H
haemangioma 121
haematoma 39, 49, 81, 147, 178
haemorrhage 49
hair, normal growth cycle 206–7
hair loss:
    assessment 201–2
    treatments 200–6
      non-surgical 205–6
      surgical 203–5
hair removal 121, 123, 206–13
    methods 207–13
hair transplantation 203–5
healing, abnormal 48
herbs, dietary 81, 231–3
herpes 110
hopes and expectations 51
hyaluronic acid 103–5
hydrocortisone 113
Hylaform 105
hymen repair 181–2
hyperhydrosis 118

I
Illouz, Dr Gerard 21, 168
implants:
    breast:
      cancer and 154
      deflation 151
      folding 150
      leakage 152
      lifespan 153
      nipple sensitivity 151–2
      problems 53
      protrusion 150–1
      rejection of 163
      removal 154
      rupture 152–3
      safety 155–7
      shape 144
      structural variations 144–5
      surface 144
      types 143–4
      wrinkling 150
    buttock 217–19
    cadaver 92, 93
    calf 214–15
    cheeks 88–90
    chest 216–17
    chin 138–40
    genital 182
    lips 92, 93
    in wrinkles 100, 108
infection 39–40, 224
injections, preoperative 65–6
intense pulsed light (IPL) 122–3, 192–3, 207–8, 213
intravenous infusion set 62

J
Jessner's solution 113, 114
jewellery, removing 65
Joseph, Jacques 130

K
keratoconjunctivitis sicca 97